Agenda for Continuing Education

A Challenge to Health Care Institutions

by

Daniel S. Schechter

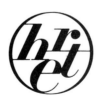

Hospital Research and Educational Trust
840 North Lake Shore Drive • Chicago, Illinois 60611

ISBN 0-87914-027-5
Library of Congress Catalog Card Number: 74-83051

© 1974 by the
Hospital Research and Educational Trust
840 North Lake Shore Drive
Chicago, Illinois 60611
All rights reserved

Printed in the U.S.A.

HRET T-36

7M—7/74—304

To Sally

Contents

FOREWORD

This foreword is responsive to my professional interests and concerns, as well as to the claims of lifelong friendship with the author. Daniel Schechter has played an important role over the last decade and more in extending the reach of the American Hospital Association into the training arena. The present modest volume is his most recent contribution to this important ongoing endeavor.

A few words about the manner in which he treats his subject, and then a few more words about where the present study fits into the large rubric of medical manpower planning and programming.

Schechter tells a straightforward tale about a new occupation: the hospital trainer—where he comes from, what he does, and how he can enhance his contribution to the efficiency of the institution and to the career development of the hospital staff. The critical themes that he adumbrates are the constructive role that a full-time education director can play in both large and small hospitals; the desirability of cooperative training programs among neighboring hospitals; the challenge to state hospital associations to take the lead in planning for cooperative programming, and assisting medical and educational centers to take professional leadership in such programming. The author also deals with the potentialities inherent in the new educational technology and stresses the importance of evaluation if continuing education is to meet the challenge it faces. This overview suggests the terrain that Schechter covers in this book.

My task is to make explicit some of the important linkages between continuing education and health manpower planning, some of which Schechter addresses briefly, others that he notes, and still others that fall outside his purview. Continuing education is clearly not an end in itself but a means to other ends:

- Improved manpower utilization

- Career development

- Improving the quality of health care

- Providing a major axis for cooperative action among health care providers

- Improved linkages between providers and consumers of health care

Let us briefly explore each of these five important objectives from the vantage of the potential contribution of continuing education.

Improved Manpower Utilization

The American people have been slow to recognize the extent to which the health services industry has grown: it now represents one of the leading sectors of the economy and is in the same league with construction, agriculture, and education. It is almost certain that total annual expenditures for health services will exceed $100 billion before 1975, and that the health care industry will offer employment for almost 4 million persons. The heart of the industry is the general hospital, because of both its use of manpower and financial resources and the critical nature of the services it renders. The hospital has a further claim to special attention. It represents one of the few centers of resource aggregation in contrast to the many small enterprise centers consisting of a single physician and a secretary or a small group-practice unit. Consequently, if the benefits of improved management are to be effectively diffused, it is essential to strengthen the hospital.

In addition, manpower utilization requires that close attention be paid to the hospital. While some of the hospital's staff have undergone long periods of professional education and training, a large part of the total work force has had only a few days, weeks, or months of training. If an arbitrary line is drawn between workers who have had more than one year's training and those who have not, approximately half of the total work force falls within the latter group.

Even without formal training, workers pick up considerable skill and knowledge on the job from their co-workers and their superiors. However, modern management has discovered that the process of skill acquisition can be speeded and improved if the pick-up approach is strengthened and reinforced by structured opportunities for workers to broaden and deepen their skills. There are no reliable data available about the sums that American industry invests annually in the training of its work force, but knowledgeable persons believe that it runs into multiple billions. Some students who have analyzed the problem of quantification believe that total training expenditures may exceed the amount spent on basic and secondary education. In the present context, all that one need specify is that the health care industry in general and the hospital in particular have, up to the present, tended to underinvest in the continuing education of their work force below the level of the physician. In light of this, we can stipulate that added investments in education and training will lead to further gains in manpower utilization.

Career Development

An effective inhouse or industry training program must always be related to job and career opportunities. It is not reasonable to encourage workers to put forth effort to broaden their knowledge and skills unless there are prospects of their benefiting from these efforts. Likewise, it is not reasonable for employers to initiate training programs that require scarce resources unless they have vacancies that cannot be filled by hiring in the open market. In short, a major goal of training should be to contribute to a better fit between the workers who are available and the work that must be done.

Today the health services industry and, particularly, the hospital represent an environment that invites expanded training for the following reasons: the nonprofessional staff is characterized by an above-average rate of turnover; certification and licensing have resulted in the balkanization of the occupational structure; union organization of hospital workers is increasing, with strong concomitant demands for expanded mobility opportunities for the work force. These unsolved manpower challenges—excessive turnover of personnel, excessive occupational differentiations, and inadequate opportunities for career progression—carry high costs and cannot be alleviated unless the personnel structure of the hospital is radically modified. If such modifications are to succeed, they can be carried out only in consonance with an expanded system of continuing education and training.

Improved Quality of Care

A final reason why more concern and effort should be directed to the training of nonprofessional personnel derives from the disadvantages of continuing to focus exclusively on the competence of the physician as the sole determinant of the quality of medical care. The United States led the world in recognizing the importance of improving the education and training of the physician, but for too long it has neglected the training of other members of the health care team, particularly those with less than a baccalaureate degree. Yet these other members can undo the work of the most skilled physician. We have no way of knowing how many patients die because of physicians' errors, and we are even more in the dark about the unnecessary deaths caused by incompetent staff. From the occasional horror story that breaks through the veil of organizational secrecy, we learn of serious and occasionally fatal errors in medication made by one or another member of the paramedical staff. Since medical care is a team undertaking, the weakest link in the chain determines the outcome. Hence, the upgrading of technicians and aides is essential if the quality of medical care is to be secured.

Cooperative Action Among Providers

In recruiting staff, most hospitals operate within a relatively narrow geographic area. This fact, when juxtaposed with high personnel turnover rates, early forced most hospitals to take on a training mission, if only to ensure a way of meeting their staffing requirements. But most hospitals undertook training activities only out of necessity, as a defensive ploy. Because nurses had to be trained, the head of the nursing department was often given the additional responsibility of ensuring that, when necessary, education and training were provided for the other members of the staff. Each hospital met its education and training requirements as well as it could, which, in most instances, was not very well.

In recent years, more and more of the basic training that hospitals had formerly undertaken on their own behalf has been moved out of the hospital, primarily to the community college, particularly for nurses and certain groups of medical technicians. In many cases, though not in all, the transfer of basic training from the hospital to the junior or senior college has led to more efficiency in the training function, as a result of gains from scale and professionalization.

Hospitals have found it difficult to cooperate with one another with respect to beds, patient flows, professional services, and ancillary services. However, both the individual hospital and the community stand to gain from increased cooperation among hospitals, which should lead to improved output at lower costs. Because of the difficulties of effecting coordination in the planning and provision of basic medical services, cooperation on the training front, where the barriers to coordination are less formidable, offers an excellent opportunity for progress. Moreover, if joint continuing education and training programs could be developed, hospitals might lose some of their suspicions and resistances to joint action on other fronts. There are indirect as well as direct benefits to be accomplished from neighborhood and communitywide planning for continuing education and training. This would reduce the pressure on the individual hospital to offer alone a farflung group of training programs that could usurp an excessive amount of its administrative and professional manpower. Cooperative programming may provide the only sensible alternative.

Improved Linkages Between Providers and Consumers

For better or worse, and probably for better, the consumer is demanding a place in the councils of the decision makers in the health arena. Moreover, physicians have been slow to understand the consequences of the fact that the average American is much better educated than his parents and grandparents, and that more and more youngsters will complete more and more years of school. Better and more education means that the patient can carry more responsibility for his own preventive and therapeutic care. But if the consumer is to respond effectively rather than emotionally to his new responsibilities, and play a larger role in the decision-making process with regard to both the planning of health care in general and his own health care in particular, he must be afforded the opportunity to become better informed about health matters. Here is a new function for the established providers, particularly the physician and the hospital. The fact that no one knows how best to respond to this challenge only adds to its importance.

We have found that continuing education and training are important in the health care field because of the contributions they can make to improved resource utilization, to staff development, to the quality of health care, to the stimulation of cooperative action among hospitals, and to helping to prepare the consumer to cope with his broadened desires and interests. In all of these matters, the hospital's role is central. The more effectively hospitals respond, the quicker the American people will be on the road to strengthening their complex and dynamic system of health care.

ELI GINZBERG, PH.D.
A. Barton Hepburn Professor of Economics
Graduate School of Business
Columbia University

ACKNOWLEDGMENTS

I have read many books in which the author expressed gratitude to a seemingly endless group of people "without whom it would not have been possible." I know now that such expressions of appreciation are real and are necessitated from a true sense of obligation and need.

The generosity of the W. K. Kellogg Foundation in support of the Hospital Continuing Education Project and of this manuscript was personified in Andrew Pattullo.

I wish especially to thank Eli Ginzberg, Ph.D., of Columbia University, for his perceptive foreword, which places my manuscript on continuing education in a larger context of national health manpower policy. A word of appreciation should be extended to Jerome P. Lysaught, Ed.D., of the University of Rochester, for his collaboration in the chapter on educational technology.

I have benefited from the work of many talented colleagues on the staff of the American Hospital Association and of the Hospital Research and Educational Trust who have joined me in examining new directions for hospital continuing education. I am particularly indebted to Thomas M. Calero, Ph.D., E. Martin Egelston, Ph.D., Herbert K. Gatzke, and Thomas M. O'Farrell. The survey of institutional training needs was accomplished only through the enthusiastic participation of the American Society for Health Manpower Education and Training and its secretary, Sharon L. Yenney. Actual conduct of the survey was undertaken by Marian S. Kessler, Alma M. Kuby, and Lorraine Richter. Patty L. McConaghey contributed greatly to the section on evaluation, as did James P. Cooney Jr., Ph.D., to the section on continuing education of hospital administrators. Colin W. Churchill and Marjorie M. Lawson have given me strong support throughout.

To my secretary, Maryann Kavanagh, and others, I am indebted for the typing of a succession of drafts.

Finally, to my wife, Sally, and to my family, who showed great patience throughout the two years of writing, I offer thanks beyond any expression of which I am capable.

DANIEL S. SCHECHTER

1

A Delivery System
for Continuing Education

January 1964 saw the start of a project designed to expand opportunities for continuing education for the personnel of health care institutions. This was the Hospital Continuing Education Project, inaugurated with a grant of $1.3 million, later supplemented by an additional $600,000, from the W. K. Kellogg Foundation to the Hospital Research and Educational Trust, an affiliate of the American Hospital Association. The purpose was to establish a new network of communication and to promote cooperation among universities, hospital associations, hospitals, and individual educators and trainers. The project, of which I was director, was carried out over nine years, terminating in 1972.

The work done under the project has created models for agencies and institutions offering continuing education. Like all such efforts, it was incomplete in itself, and was not expected to be otherwise. I believe that it offers some useful leads, and some signs that people of good will can really work productively together for the benefit of those to whom they are all dedicated in service.

Many basic questions still require study: Exactly what constitutes continuing education? How should a hospital define the extent and the limits of its educational commitment? What is the responsibility of members of the professions for their own continuing education? What is the best learning environment for administrators, department managers, supervisors, professional employees, or other categories of hospital personnel? How can programs be evaluated? What kinds of effort are needed from hospital associations, educational institutions, government agencies, private industry? What are presently the most urgent needs in the field of hospital-oriented continuing education?

ACTIVITIES OF THE HOSPITAL CONTINUING EDUCATION PROJECT

The staff of the Hospital Continuing Education Project tried to make clear to the persons and agencies who participated in the project that we would not evaluate activities on the traditional basis of the number of persons who attended educational programs. For too long this has been the measure of success in adult education, both in and out of the health care field. Rather, we were interested in their developing the type of programming that was most needed and that each participating agency was uniquely equipped to offer. We did not want universities performing like hospital associations, nor the other way around. What we did want was to find a way of linking universities and hospital associations, the better to serve hospital personnel.

The project actually was carried out as a group of experimental activities, or sub-projects, related to the following specific goals:

1. To develop collaborative programs between health care institutions and educational institutions
2. To promote and experiment with hospitalwide educational programs managed by a director of education and training
3. To facilitate the preparation of persons to administer or teach in continuing education programs
4. To encourage educators to conduct regional needs analyses
5. To sponsor experimentation in the uses of educational technology

One part of the project that we planned to be of immediate use to hospital-based educators and trainers was the publication, *Training and Continuing Education: A Handbook for Health Care Institutions* (Chicago: Hospital Research and Educational Trust, 1970), a practical guide to theory and techniques, with copious samples of teaching materials. Other publications resulting from the project dealt with nursing service management, with correspondence education, and with university centers for hospital continuing education.

University Centers for Continuing Education

One of our major goals was to put hospitals in touch with the resources of community colleges and universities. Between 1964 and 1966 the Hospital Research and Educational Trust opened experimental regional centers for continuing education for hospital personnel in seven universities, all of which had graduate programs in hospital administration and therefore had already demonstrated their commitment to the health care field.[1] The universities were: University of Alabama, University of California, Columbia University, Duke University, University of Michigan, University of Minnesota, and St. Louis University.

Our thesis was that universities, in addition to their functions of undergraduate and graduate education and research, have an obligation to public service compatible with their interests, and that universities with hospital administration programs could demonstrate that responsibility by offering continuing education to health care personnel.

---

1. Daniel S. Schechter and Thomas M. O'Farrell, *Universities, Colleges, and Hospitals: Partners in Continuing Education* (Battle Creek, Mich.: W. K. Kellogg Foundation, 1972).

We hoped that each of these universities would become a center of creative programming and coordination of hospital continuing education in its geographical region.

The programs of the university centers, like all other programs sponsored by the Hospital Continuing Education Project, were nonclinical and focused on improving hospital management. The reader will note that this book, which presumes to deal with "hospital continuing education," omits specific treatment of continuing medical education and the major role and responsibilities of the hospital in facilitating it. Other authors have written knowledgeably on that subject. It should be noted that the chapters dealing with university centers (Chapter 4) and with hospitalwide education and training (Chapter 3) suggest a framework in which continuing education for both physicians and others can be approached.

Residential–Home-Study Programs

Along with the development of the university centers, the project staff decided to experiment with university-based courses in hospital administration that combined short periods of on-campus instruction with home study. Six universities cooperated with us by offering such courses to administrators of smaller hospitals and, in some cases, of nursing homes, who had no graduate training in hospital administration. We were more successful in enticing state universities than private institutions into trying this format because they recognized their community service role, because they already had extension departments, and also because they were not so worried about what would happen to their reputations if they offered courses that (whether so labeled or not) had as a major element "home study."

Between 1965 and 1970, the Hospital Continuing Education Project inaugurated "residential-home-study" programs at the University of Alabama; University of California; Trinity University, San Antonio, Texas; University of Minnesota; and Ohio State University. In addition, the project assisted the program at Columbia University, started earlier under a separate grant from the W. K. Kellogg Foundation.

State Association Directors of Education

We also invited a limited number of state and regional hospital associations to work with the Hospital Continuing Education Project and with their member hospitals to foster hospitalwide continuing education. These associations are close to the individual hospitals the project was to serve, and the staff felt that perhaps the best way to strengthen educational programs in individual institutions was to work through the persons in state and regional organizations who had responsibility for education and training. The problem was that there were almost no such positions in existence in associations, and all too few in hospitals. Our plan was to enable the state and regional associations working with us to employ directors of education who would promote continuing education on a statewide basis, at a district level within their states, and also within individual hospitals.

When we started, only three state hospital associations employed professional educators, either part or full time. We claim considerable credit for the fact that when the project ended, there were 45 directors of education in such organizations. We hoped that the project's assistance to metropolitan, state, and regional hospital associations would complement the regional university centers program, and that these associations would be enabled to make good use of the resources offered by the university centers.

During 1966-68, three-year grants toward the support of the position of director of education were made by the Hospital Continuing Education Project to the state hospital associations of Arizona, Arkansas, Delaware, Florida, Iowa, Louisiana, Ohio (to work with the Greater Cleveland Hospital Council), Virginia, and Wisconsin, and to the New England Hospital Assembly. Throughout this three-year program, the project staff worked closely with these associations. From the outset, the American Hospital Association had intended to continue services for which a need was indicated. When grant support ended, the executive directors of the participating associations concurred in requesting that the services provided by project staff be made available to all allied associations, specifically mentioning conferences, new educational materials and programs developed and published by the American Hospital Association and the Hospital Research and Educational Trust, and informational bulletins that evaluated materials and programs available from other organizations and commercial firms.

As a result, both the American Hospital Association and the Hospital Research and Educational Trust have revised their educational programs to complement and support those of allied associations. The American Hospital Association has committed budget and staff to sponsor annual conferences and to provide services for the directors of education of all hospital associations.

Needs Determination and Technology Applications

Several other activities of the Hospital Continuing Education Project were concentrated in two areas to which we felt that the hospital field had given too little attention: the determination of need for training and education and the application of technology to the process of education and training.

Too many educational programs in the health care field have been undertaken without sufficient indication that they were addressed to real needs. We urged all recipients of grants from the project to make surveys of needs before setting up programs, and we supported a number of regional and state surveys of the educational needs of administrative and supervisory personnel, which furnished data for several of the programs of university centers and allied associations.

The second relatively neglected area was experimentation with new educational methods and technology. It seemed to us that programmed instruction, to take one example, might be useful for extending the effectiveness of hospital instructors who might be expert practitioners but might have had little training expertise. To explore this area of educational technology, the Clearinghouse on Self-Instructional Materials for Health Care Facilities was established by the project in 1966 at the University of Rochester (New York). Operating under the auspices of the School of Medicine and Dentistry, with the cooperation of the College of Education, the Clearinghouse had the following functions:

1. To collect information on self-instructional materials for use in the hospital by nonprofessional members of the hospital staff

2. To publish information about these materials in a brief newsletter with bibliographic citations

3. To respond to queries from hospitals about specific programs

4. To offer facilities for examination of both materials and teaching devices

Hospitalwide Education and Training

To further assist individual hospitals the Hospital Continuing Education Project conducted during 1969-70 a series of 11 regional conferences attended by approximately 1000 persons designated by their hospitals as currently or potentially responsible for hospitalwide education and training.

When the project began in 1964, few hospitals had hospitalwide training programs. Not many directors of medical education were extending their sights beyond the needs of interns, residents, and other physicians. Most existing training programs were administered by nurses for nurses, or by personnel specialists who sought assistance with training and were frequently not sure of their own roles. Many of the persons who attended the conferences in 1969-70 suggested that the American Hospital Association establish a permanent organization that could offer assistance and serve as a forum for them. As a result, in September 1970, the Board of Trustees of the American Hospital Association authorized a new personal membership society, the American Society for Health Manpower Education and Training.

Twenty-five local chapters had affiliated with the society by the end of 1973, and the roster of individual members listed over 1200 names. About one-third of these members were directors of hospitalwide education and training and, significantly, another one-third were nursing inservice education personnel. Other members were faculty of colleges, universities, and hospital schools of nursing; directors of medical education; public health personnel; and hospital administrators. The society now serves as the professional organization for educators concerned with the development and continuing education of hospital and other health care personnel.

NEED FOR A DELIVERY SYSTEM

During the last decade, while professional and public attention was focused on improving the delivery of health care services, the Hospital Continuing Education Project was concerned with a parallel need, the need for creating an educational delivery system, forging agreement and commitment among the many organizations and institutions interested in optimal use of health manpower. Nothing less than such a system will satisfy personnel development needs, institutional service needs, and public expectations and demands.

Many of these needs were identified through our experience with the Hospital Continuing Education Project and were further clarified and documented through the survey of members of the American Society for Health Manpower Education and Training, described in the next chapter. In succeeding chapters I will discuss some of these needs in detail and put forward some specific proposals for meeting them.

2

National Survey of
Hospital-Based Trainers

To take an organized look at both institutional training and educational needs in such a rapidly changing field, and at the personal development needs of those doing the training within hospitals, a long series of questions was posed to the members of the American Society for Health Manpower Education and Training who were actually on the firing line of hospital educational programming in 1972.

The survey was designed to provide data on the background, experience, and formal preparation of these educators and trainers, with explanations of where and how they fit into the organizational structure of the health care institutions in which they work. Additionally, the responses tell what job activities they performed and what methods they employ. The trainers were asked to venture predictions for the future in terms of training needs in hospitals and of their own needs for professional development.

The findings from this survey provide a firm basis for describing what those actually involved with the educational and training process in health care institutions think is needed.

There were 640 responses to the survey, representing nearly 70 percent of the membership of the American Society for Health Manpower Education and Training, which totaled more than 900 in December 1971. However, 104 responses (about one-sixth) were from members not directly affiliated with health care providers but engaged in activities in related fields—42 percent in higher education of health personnel, 27 percent in state hospital associations, and the remainder in such areas as the allied health professions, Regional Medical Programs, and health careers recruitment. These members were asked to answer only five basic questions.

The other five-sixths of the respondents, the 536 persons working as educators and trainers in health care institutions at the time of the survey, completed all of the detailed questions in the 14-page questionnaire and provided the information that is the basis for this discussion.

The excellent response reflected not only the generous cooperation of these trainers, but the value of the questionnaire in aiding them to define their activities and their needs, and to plan more effectively. Others engaged in planning educational programs may find it helpful to review this survey instrument (Appendix A).

HOSPITALS EMPLOYING TRAINERS

Trainers are employed by hospitals in all census division regions of the United States, with the greatest numbers located in the Middle Atlantic and East North Central states (Table 1, next page). (For the sake of brevity, "trainers" will be used here to mean those who identify themselves as trainers or educators.) Forty-five percent of the trainers work in cities classified by the 1970 census as the 100 largest cities in the United States. Inasmuch as only 19 percent of the nation's hospitals are located in these cities, trainers are highly concentrated in large urban centers.

Since the number of specialized services requiring highly trained technical personnel increases with hospital size, and the larger hospitals are predominantly found in metropolitan areas, it is not surprising that less than a quarter of the respondents were employed by hospitals having fewer than 200 beds, although hospitals of this size constitute over 70 percent of the nation's hospitals.

Location of the Training Function in the Organization

As one might expect, separate departments of education are found mostly in large hospitals; in small hospitals with fewer departments, the training function is frequently located in the departments of nursing, for nursing has a long history of inservice education and training (Table 2, next page). Fifty-two percent of the respondents reported that their hospitals maintain separate departments for hospitalwide training activities; however, it is unclear whether the term "hospitalwide" conveyed the same meaning to all respondents, since of these departments, one-third were called departments of nursing education; 28 percent were called departments of education; and 39 percent were staff development, personnel, and other administrative departments. About half of all respondents were working in nursing service or nursing education departments, 15 percent in education departments, and the remainder in administrative and personnel departments.[1] In hospitals with fewer than 200 beds, about two-thirds of the respondents were affiliated with nursing departments, and only a few with departments of education; and in hospitals with fewer than 100 beds, 28 of the 37 respondents were in departments of nursing. On the other hand, of the respondents

---

1. Similar findings were obtained in an earlier survey of hospital manpower and training in 203 New England hospitals, conducted in 1969-70 for the New England Hospital Assembly by the New England Center for Continuing Education, University of New Hampshire. Only 9 percent of those hospitals then employed a hospital training director. Training responsibilities rested with the nursing director in 73 percent of the hospitals surveyed, with the personnel department in 45 percent, and with department heads in 26 percent.

Table 1. Distribution of Respondents by Region and by Hospital Size

Region	Hospital Size (Beds)							
	All Sizes	Under 100	100-199	200-299	300-399	400-499	500 and over	Not Specified
All regions	536	37	88	103	93	77	133	5
New England	35	4	10	5	6	7	3	—
Middle Atlantic	101	7	16	22	16	11	29	—
South Atlantic	76	6	11	16	12	11	18	2
East North Central	145	5	22	17	30	25	43	3
East South Central	20	1	2	4	5	2	6	—
West North Central	56	4	9	13	7	9	14	—
West South Central	35	1	7	9	6	6	6	—
Mountain	25	3	3	6	5	3	5	—
Pacific	43	6	8	11	6	3	9	—

Table 2. Distribution of Respondents by Hospital Size and by Departmental Location

Hospital Size (Beds)	All Departments (N=536)	Nursing (N=262)	Education (N=82)	Other* (N=192)
All sizes	100%	100%	100%	100%
Under 100	7	11	5	3
100-199	17	20	7	15
200-299	19	22	20	16
300-399	17	16	28	14
400-499	14	13	12	18
500 and over	25	17	28	33
Not specified	1	1	—	1

*Includes personnel, administration, and staff development.

from departments of education or administrative departments, more than two-thirds were employed by hospitals with 300 or more beds.

Respondents from large hospitals reported that in addition to their own training activities, training programs were developed in other departments. A considerable number of clinical training programs were run by clinical departments (medical staff and laboratory and medical records) and some hospitalwide trainers reported that specialized training programs were developed and conducted within nursing units.

In an attempt to see whether departmental affiliation influences trainers' techniques, programs, or views on professional and institutional needs, some of the survey information will be discussed with reference to its departmental context.

CHARACTERISTICS OF TRAINERS

Three of every four respondents were women. Nearly one-third of the trainers were between 40 and 49 years of age, and an equal proportion were a decade younger. Only eight respondents (one percent) were under 25 years of age, and 13 percent were

Table 3. Distribution of Respondents by Age and Sex

Age and Sex	Number	Percent
All respondents	536	100
Age		
Under 25 years	8	1
25-29	71	13
30-39	167	32
40-49	169	32
50-59	103	19
60 and over	12	2
Not specified	6	1
Sex		
Male	134	25
Female	401	75
Not specified	1	—

in their late twenties. The remaining 21 percent were over 50 (Table 3, above).

The breadth of professional interests and the extent of schooling of these hospital-based trainers are impressive. Thirty-six percent held advanced degrees at the master's level or above, three percent having the M.D. or Ph.D.; and an additional 36 percent had bachelor's degrees (Table 4, next page). The range of their formal studies encompassed nursing (21 percent), education (14 percent), nursing education (10 percent), and administration (9 percent). Those who earned master's or doctoral degrees had specialized in guidance, administration, or education. Other fields included liberal arts, personnel, science, and technology. Among respondents were four physicians, a chaplain, a journalist, and an environmentalist. Twenty-six percent of the respondents indicated no college degree.

It is clear that those now charged with training responsibilities in the area of health manpower are well schooled, but, for the most part, not in the field of education. Only about one-tenth of the respondents had earned teaching certificates; most of the group held credentials in nursing.

Work Experience

As a group, the survey respondents showed considerable experience in the health care field, but the majority (65 percent) had been in their current positions for less than three years (Table 5, next page). Twenty-eight percent of the respondents in education departments and 15 percent of those in nursing departments had held their current positions for less than one year.

Trainers in education departments were more likely to have had previous experience in training and education than trainers in nursing departments. Thirty-one percent of the nursing department respondents reported having had no training experience prior to their current positions, in contrast to approximately half that proportion (16 percent) of the education department group. Fifty-six percent of the education department trainers, but only 33 percent of the nursing department respondents, reported five or more years of previous experience as trainers. On the other hand, fewer educa-

Table 4. Distribution of Respondents by Educational Background

Educational Background	Number	Percent
All respondents	536	100
Highest degree		
Associate	12	2
Bachelor	191	36
Master's	177	33
Doctorate	15	3
None or no answer	141	26
Field of degree		
Nursing Education	52	10
Nursing	113	21
Education	73	14
Guidance	12	2
Personnel	7	1
Administration	49	9
Medicine	4	1
Medical Technology	17	3
Other Science	25	5
Liberal Arts	35	7
Other, area unknown	8	1
None	141	26

Table 5. Distribution of Respondents by Specified Experience
and by Departmental Location

Experience	Department		
	All Departments (*N*=536)	Nursing (*N*=262)	Education (*N*=82)
All respondents	100%	100%	100%
Prior employment in health care field			
None	13	1	23
Less than 1 year	2	4	4
1 to 3 years	9	7	11
3 to 5 years	7	7	6
5 years or more	69	81	56
Prior experience as trainer/educator			
None	25	31	16
Less than 1 year	6	7	6
1 to 3 years	16	17	12
3 to 5 years	12	12	10
5 years or more	41	33	56
Present employment as trainer/educator			
Less than 1 year	19	15	28
1 to 3 years	46	45	43
3 to 5 years	19	20	21
5 years or more	16	20	8

tion department trainers had been previously employed in the health care field.

The diverse academic backgrounds of the respondents have already been noted. It is obvious that this diversity is amplified by the variety in the type and extent of previous employment, and further complicated by the relatively short time the respondents had held their current assignments. These factors should be kept in mind as the survey findings are reviewed.

DETERMINING TRAINING NEEDS

The survey investigated the trainers' use of six different methods of assessing institutional training needs: interviews with administrators and with department heads and supervisors, questionnaire surveys of employee groups, work studies of employee performance, analysis of records and informal conversations (Table 6, next page). All these methods were used by the respondents; each was mentioned by 60 percent or more of the respondents in connection with assessing at least one institutional need.

In addition to using more than one method of assessing needs before making decisions on projected activities, trainers attempted coordination; before committing themselves to programs concerned with orientation, continuing education, supervisory development, and interdepartmental coordination, 85 percent or more of the respondents interviewed the supervisors and department heads concerned. Respondents who planned or conducted programs in the areas specified in the survey indicated that these interviews, together with informal conversations, were the methods they most frequently used to determine training needs. On the other hand, in determining needs in the areas of upper management development, medical staff continuing education, and community health education, interviews with administrative personnel were primary.

Respondents used hard data from employee questionnaires, performance evaluations, and records analysis to some extent in determining training needs, most often to assess needs for entry-level skills training and for continuing education. However, this approach apparently has neither the appeal nor the effectiveness of interviews and informal conversation. It is possible, of course, that the respondents' preference resulted from their inexperience with hard-data techniques.

PLANNING AND CONDUCTING PROGRAMS

The programming activities of the respondents were measured through their reports of programs they had planned or conducted to meet specific training needs (Table 7, next page). Planning or conducting orientation programs for new employees was their most common activity, reported by 85 percent of the trainers. Continuing education and entry-level skills training were also high on the list of activities planned or conducted by trainers. Possible training needs least likely to have received attention by hospital trainers were those of the medical staff or those of employees with literacy deficiencies.

Trainers planned more programs than they conducted, although most respondents reported having done both. Nineteen percent of the respondents had personally planned or conducted programs in four of the training needs areas listed in the survey; 17 percent in more than six areas; and a few respondents reported having planned or conducted programs in all 12 areas.

Table 6. Percent of Respondents Using Specified Methods to Determine
Training/Education Needs for Programs Planned or Conducted

Training/Education Need for Which Programs Were Planned or Conducted	Number Conducting or Planning Programs	Percent of Respondents Using Specified Method				
		Interviews with:		Surveys of Employee Groups	Performance Studies & Record Analysis	Informal Conver- sation
		Adminis- tration	Dept. Heads & Super- visors			
Orientation	453	54	87	47	55	82
Entry-level skills training	386	32	81	37	61	67
Continuing education	398	47	86	62	57	76
Refresher training	250	37	71	33	43	60
Upper management development ..	194	85	69	38	32	53
Supervisory development	293	66	85	42	38	58
Medical staff continuing education .	42	50	36	14	12	48
Interdepartmental coordination	172	64	87	27	20	58
Community health education	123	62	47	13	13	54
Patient education	159	35	75	19	23	—
Basic literacy training	56	29	57	32	16	27
English as second language	35	40	60	17	20	37

Table 7. Percent of Respondents Reporting Programs Planned or Conducted to Meet
Specified Training/Education Needs, by Departmental Location of Respondent

Training/Education Need	All Departments* (N=536)	Nursing (N=262)	Education (N=82)
Orientation	85%	89%	77%
Entry-level skills training	72	84	71
Continuing education	74	87	61
Refresher training	47	53	46
Upper management development	36	24	56
Supervisory development	55	45	65
Medical staff continuing education	8	6	17
Interdepartmental coordination	32	28	37
Community health education	23	23	28
Patient education	30	37	29
Basic literacy training	10	3	16
English as second language	7	3	9

*Includes 192 respondents in departments other than nursing and education, including administration, personnel, and staff development.

Differences in the kinds of programming most frequently planned or conducted appear to be related to the trainers' departmental affiliations. Nursing department trainers reported more activity in the areas of orientation, entry-level skills training, continuing education, refresher training, and patient education. Education department trainers reported more activity in the areas of upper management and supervisory development, medical staff continuing education, interdepartmental coordination, community health education, and basic literacy training.

Participants in Training Programs

More training activities are planned and conducted for nurses than for any other group in hospitals (Table 8, next page). Eighty-eight percent of the respondents reported having planned or conducted programs for nurses within the previous 12 months. Training programs for supportive personnel, including dietary and house-keeping employees and volunteers, were reported by 73 percent of the respondents. Programs for administrative personnel and department heads were reported by 61 percent, and for clinical staff by 53 percent.

Many trainers, whether affiliated with nursing departments, education departments, or other departments, reported having planned or conducted programs for all types of participant groups. However, less than half of the nursing department respondents reported having planned or conducted programs for administrators, department heads, and clinical staff; rather, they tended to concentrate on activities for nursing personnel. More than three-quarters of the education department respondents reported having planned or conducted programs for all categories of participants. Trainers affiliated with staff development, personnel, or other administrative departments reported less involvement with clinical staff (medical staff and laboratory and medical records personnel). Thus, it appears that education department trainers are more likely to have responsibility and authority for planning and conducting hospitalwide training.

Cooperative and Shared Training Programs

Today it is not uncommon for hospitals to provide training programs in cooperation with educational institutions and with other hospitals (Table 9, next page). About four-fifths of the respondents reported that their hospitals conducted degree or certificate programs in cooperation with educational institutions. This proportion obtained throughout the country, with only slight regional variations. Vocational-technical schools cooperated in programming (especially for nurses and clinical aides) with hospitals represented by 44 percent of the respondents. Nearly as many respondents reported cooperative programming with junior colleges (42 percent) and with universities (40 percent). High schools, four-year colleges, and other institutions also participated with the respondents' hospitals in training programs.

A smaller but still sizable number of respondents (57 percent) reported that their hospitals shared health manpower training programs with other health care institutions. Most of these programs were planned as career training for graduate nurses. Thirty-two percent of the respondents reported that their hospitals were cooperating with other health care centers in graduate nurse training programs; 18 percent indicated that there would be additional or new cooperative programs under way by 1974. Sixteen percent of the respondents reported that their hospitals had shared training programs for licensed practical nurses, and 8 percent were planning such programs. Other popular shared training programs were those for allied health technologists and aides and for administrative personnel.

It is interesting to compare these figures on shared training programs with those obtained from a national survey of shared services conducted in July 1971 by the Health Services Research Center of the Hospital Research and Educational Trust and Northwestern University, in cooperation with the American Hospital Association's

Table 8. Percent of Respondents Reporting Programs Planned or Conducted for Specified Participant Groups, by Departmental Location of Respondent

Participant Group	All Departments (N=536)	Nursing (N=262)	Education (N=82)	Other* (N=192)
Nursing personnel	88%	96%	79%	80%
Supportive personnel (includes dietary, housekeeping, and volunteer)	73	70	79	74
Administrative and departmental personnel (includes administration, department heads, and supervisors)	61	44	82	76
Clinical personnel (includes medical staff, laboratory, and medical records)	53	41	77	58

*Includes administration, personnel, and staff development.

Table 9. Distribution of Respondents Reporting Cooperative Programs with Educational Institutions, and with Other Health Care Institutions, by Type of Institution and by Type of Program Participant

Type of Institution and of Program Participant	Number	Percent
All respondents	536	100
Programs with educational institutions	435	80
University	220	40
Four-year college	139	26
Junior college	231	42
Vocational-technical school	238	44
High school	118	22
Other	58	11
Programs with other health care institutions	306	57
Graduate nurses	174	32
Licensed practical nurses	88	16
Allied health technologists	53	10
Administrative personnel	48	9
Allied health aides	47	9
Undergraduate nurses	32	6
Medical staff	30	6
All other	62	11

Bureau of Research Services.[2] In that survey, the percentage of hospital administrators reporting shared nursing inservice programs (both current and projected) was smaller than the percentage of hospital-based trainers reporting such programs in the survey under discussion here. Considerations of survey error aside, it appears that the proportion of respondents' hospitals with shared programs is greater than the proportion of all hospitals with such programs. One must therefore raise the question of whether the presence of a trainer precedes the development of shared programs, or whether

---

2. See *AHA Fact Survey Sheet—No. 7* (Chicago: American Hospital Association, Bureau of Research Services, July 1972), and "Survey profiles shared services," by Adrienne A. Astolfi and Leo P. Matti, *Hospitals, J.A.H.A.*, 46:61, Sept. 16, 1972.

Table 10. Percent of Respondents Reporting Specified Programming Items as Staff-Developed or from Commercial Sources

Programming Item	Percent Reporting (N = 536)	
	Staff-Developed	Commercial Sources
Educational TV (outside channels)	—	22
Closed circuit TV	23	15
Slide-sound presentations	42	47
Filmstrips	8	74
Filmstrip-sound presentations	7	79
Transparencies	69	35
8mm movies	5	19
16mm movies	7	86
Tape recordings (audio)	55	45
Cassette tapes (audio)	53	55
Case problems	53	24
Demonstrations	83	28
Role plays	60	12
Training games	25	17
Action mazes	3	4
In-basket exercises	18	19
Sensitivity training exercises	15	8
Programmed instruction materials	21	62
Instructor's guides	39	65
Student manuals	42	57
Lesson plans	76	24
Evaluation questionnaires or rating forms	84	22

existing shared programs mushroom beyond the capabilities of departmental personnel and necessitate the employment of a professional trainer.

Hospital trainers draw on outside resources not only for cooperative programming but also for training programs within the hospital. During the 12-month period preceding the survey, 89 percent of the respondents invited speakers or instructors from outside their institutions to assist in training programs, and 46 percent obtained the services of outside consultants to assist with program development in specialized fields.

Educational Methods and Materials

Hospital-based trainers are aware of, and are using, an extensive variety of educational methods and materials. Of 22 items of educational hardware and software listed in the survey questionnaire, most of the respondents favored seven or eight types of materials from commercial sources and an equal number of types of different items developed by themselves or by their staffs (Table 10, above). Most trainers had relied on their own staff-developed evaluation forms, demonstrations, and lesson plans. Well over half of the respondents had also devised their role-playing situations and had produced transparencies, audio cassettes, and tapes. As to purchased items, more than three-quarters of all respondents had bought movies, filmstrips, and filmstrip-sound presentations. A majority of the respondents had also invested in commercially prepared instructors' guides, student manuals, and programmed instruction materials, and in audio cassettes.

Table 11. Percent of Respondents Reporting Specified Items of Audiovisual Equipment as Available or Planned

Item of Equipment	Percent Reporting (*N* = 536)	
	Now Available	Plan to Purchase
Overhead projector	86	4
Opaque projector	59	4
Slide projector	92	3
Filmstrip projector	87	4
8mm movie projector	24	2
16mm movie projector	95	1
Tape recorder (reel)	77	1
Cassette recorder	79	7
Cassette tape player	73	5
TV camera	34	7
Still camera	49	4
8mm movie camera	12	3
16mm movie camera	15	2
Slide-tape synchronizer	26	7
Videotape recorder	37	9
Videotape player	41	9

In regard to audiovisual equipment, almost all respondents reported having on hand a 16mm projector and a slide projector (Table 11, above). Most respondents also had overhead and filmstrip projectors in their hospitals. Tape and cassette recorders and players were available to most trainers as well. A query about plans for future purchases evoked nearly all negative responses; the highest proportion of positive responses (9 percent) came from those planning to buy videotape equipment.

Budgets for Training

Budgetary constraints doubtless enter into considerations of what materials to purchase. Although 57 percent of the respondents stated that the dollar amounts available to them for training activities had increased in the past two years (Table 12, page 18), only 15 percent had a current budget that approached an ideal figure (Table 13, page 18). The greatest increases in available funds were reported by trainers in hospital education departments, 39 percent of whom reported a significant growth. Eleven percent of the respondents indicated no change in funding for training activities in the past two years, and reductions in funds were reported by 7 percent.

Respondents were asked to measure their current funds against ideal budgets that would meet all their needs. Ten percent of the respondents reported that their current funds were less than 10 percent of what their ideal budgets would be. Of those indicating that their actual budgets were less than half of the ideal, only 24 percent were in education departments, in contrast to 40 percent in nursing departments and 45 percent in other departments.

Almost one-quarter of the respondents failed to answer this question, possibly because of fiscal inexperience, or of concern over publicizing financial information. However, many respondents expressed their budgetary concerns indirectly. For example, in one question respondents were asked to estimate the degree of their influence

Table 12. Percent of Respondents Reporting Specified Changes in Availability of Training Funds During Past Two Years, by Departmental Location

Change in Availability of Funds	All Departments (N=536)	Nursing (N=262)	Education (N=82)	Other* (N=192)
All respondents	100%	100%	100%	100%
Grown significantly	29	24	39	30
Grown somewhat	28	28	26	29
Stayed the same	11	13	9	10
Been reduced somewhat	5	4	5	6
Been reduced significantly	2	2	0	3
No funds allocated to training/education	10	12	8	7
Other (includes "no records," no answer, and other)	15	17	13	15

*Includes administration, personnel, and staff development.

Table 13. Percent of Respondents Comparing Actual Training Funds to Specified Percentages of "Ideal Budget" That Would Meet All Training Needs

Actual Funds as Percent of Ideal Budget	All Departments (N=536)	Nursing (N=262)	Education (N=82)	Other* (N=192)
All respondents	100%	100%	100%	100%
Less than 10 percent	10	10	4	15
10 - 25 percent	12	13	9	11
26 - 50 percent	17	17	11	19
51 - 75 percent	23	21	37	19
76 - 100 percent	15	12	19	16
No answer	23	27	20	20

*Includes administration, personnel, and staff development.

in "acquiring needed funds for activities"; most trainers indicated that they believed they had only moderate or little influence, and 10 percent indicated that the question was not relevant to their jobs.

Budgetary concerns also were expressed in response to another question that focused on problems encountered by trainers in their work. Insufficient budget and too few qualified personnel were problems indicated by more than half of the respondents. (Inability to recruit staff may be, but is not necessarily, a consequence of budget shortcomings.) In answer to still another question, more than half of the respondents expressed a desire for additional information about measuring the costs of training.

TRAINERS' PERCEPTIONS OF THEIR JOBS

Influence Over Specified Job Components

Respondents were asked to estimate the degree of influence they exercised over each of nine listed components of their jobs (Table 14, next page). At least 60 percent reported a high degree of influence in five categories: determining needs, setting objectives, determining content, selecting instructors, and evaluating programs. Most of the remaining respondents described themselves as having moderate influence in these areas, with less than 10 percent reporting low influence.

Table 14. Distribution of Respondents by Their Designated Estimates of Their Degree of Influence Over Specified Job Components

Job Component	All respondents (N=536)	Degree of Influence			
		High	Moderate	Low	Not Relevant
Setting training and educational objectives	100%	76%	21%	2%	2%
Determining content	100	73	23	2	2
Determining training and educational needs	100	69	27	2	2
Selecting speakers and instructors	100	68	23	4	5
Evaluating the results of programs	100	63	28	5	4
Selecting program participants or trainees	100	46	39	10	5
Supervising programs carried out by others	100	35	33	18	14
Developing programs to be carried out by others	100	33	39	17	11
Acquiring needed funds for activities	100	26	39	25	10

Less than half of the respondents reported having high influence over the remaining categories of job components: selecting participant groups, developing or supervising programs to be carried out by others, and acquiring funds. Since no more than 14 percent of the respondents designated any one of these items as not relevant to their jobs, it would appear that some trainers require further assistance in these areas.

Differences in influence over job components are apparent when one compares the responses of nursing department trainers to the responses of education department trainers (Table 15, page 21). The nursing group reported more influence in determining content, selecting instructors, and designating program participants, but the education group indicated slightly more influence over setting objectives, determining needs, supervising and developing programs for others, and acquiring funds. Perhaps these differences can be explained by the fact that nursing department trainers focus on their more specific assignments, while education department trainers focus on hospitalwide training.

Problems Encountered

Trainers see the problems that impede effective performance of their duties as institutional rather than personal. In response to a list of seven problems that they might encounter in carrying out their duties, over half of the respondents indicated that a shortage of qualified personnel and inadequate budget are the most troublesome (Table 16, page 21). Only 28 percent identified personal deficiencies in knowledge or skills as a problem.

There are some interesting variations among the responses classified by departments. For example, trainers in nursing and in "other" (including administration, personnel, and staff development) departments appear to have less access to higher administrative personnel than do trainers in education departments; 49 percent of the nursing department trainers and 44 percent of those in "other" departments reported that there was not enough involvement on the part of higher management, in contrast to 29 percent of the education department trainers. More nursing and "other" department respondents than education department respondents indicated that they had insufficient authority to make decisions. Also, inadequate preparation for training functions was acknowledged by more "other" department trainers (41 percent) and nursing department trainers (37 percent) than education department trainers (21 percent).

The two problems ranked highest for all departments were, first, not enough qualified staff and, second, insufficient budget. These were problems for a majority of all respondents and for at least half of those classified by departments. Further exploration would be required to evaluate the significance of these responses.

Learning Needs of Trainers

With what aspects of their jobs might hospital-based trainers welcome assistance? The survey questionnaire enumerated nine aspects of a trainer's work, asking respondents to check those about which they would like to know more. These nine aspects may be classified as follows:

PROGRAM PLANNING
1. Assessing training needs
2. Setting measurable objectives

PROGRAM IMPLEMENTATION
3. Building learning principles into program designs
4. Combining elements of an educational program effectively
5. Achieving an effective instructional methods "mix"

PROGRAMMING MATERIALS
6. Creating training materials (e.g., course outlines, workbooks)
7. Evaluating packaged programs available from outside sources

EVALUATION
8. Evaluating training programs within the institution

COSTS
9. Measuring training and nontraining costs

The respondents, taken as a whole, expressed most interest in additional information about evaluation of inhouse training programs (Table 17, page 22).[3] Sixty-three percent of all respondents indicated a need for learning more about evaluation of inhouse programs. Three aspects of training—measuring costs, evaluating packaged programs from outside sources, and creating training materials—ranked next; they were checked as learning needs by 51 percent of all respondents.

The number of aspects most frequently checked (by 22 percent of the respondents) was four of the possible nine (Table 18, page 22). Nine percent of the respondents expressed interest in all nine aspects.

---

3. A 1969 survey of the needs of hospital-based trainers in the southeastern United States, conducted by the Division of Health Services Administration, School of Community and Allied Health Resources, University of Alabama, also gave highest priority to the evaluation of training programs. Ranked second was how to establish management-supervisory development programs. In response to the needs elicited by this survey, a curriculum was developed for training trainers in two sessions of several days each.

Table 15. Percent of Respondents Designating a High Degree of Influence Over Specified Job Components, by Departmental Location

Job Component	Respondents Designating a High Degree of Influence			
	All Departments (*N*=536)	Nursing (*N*=262)	Education (*N*=82)	Other* (*N*=192)
Setting training and educational objectives	76%	75%	79%	76%
Determining content	73	80	65	67
Determining training and educational needs	69	69	72	69
Selecting speakers and instructors	68	74	60	65
Evaluating the results of programs	63	62	62	64
Selecting program participants or trainees	46	47	39	49
Supervising programs carried out by others	35	34	37	36
Developing programs to be carried out by others	33	31	37	36
Acquiring funds for activities	26	17	41	31

*Includes respondents in administration, personnel, and staff development.

Table 16. Percent of Respondents Designating Specified Problems Encountered in Training/Education, by Departmental Location

Problem	All Departments (*N*=536)	Nursing (*N*=262)	Education (*N*=82)	Other* (*N*=192)
Not having enough qualified people to do the work	60%	60%	50%	63%
Not having enough budget for materials, equipment, or facilities	52	55	51	49
Not getting enough involvement on the part of higher management	44	49	29	44
Not getting enough cooperation from other departments	43	42	44	43
Not having enough authority to make decisions	37	39	24	41
Not having enough outside resources available	29	32	27	27
Not having the knowledge or skills to carry out the work with confidence ...	28	37	21	19

*Includes respondents in administration, personnel, and staff development.

The 77 trainers who registered interest in only one or two of the nine aspects of training showed a high concentration on two closely related categories: measuring costs (35 percent) and evaluating inhouse training programs (30 percent) (Table 19, page 23). For trainers who indicated need for more information about three of the aspects of training these rankings were reversed: 58 percent of the 103 respondents designated evaluating inhouse training programs and 44 percent, measuring costs; while 44 percent also designated evaluation of packaged programs from outside sources.

Table 17. Percent of Respondents Indicating Desire to Know More About Specified Aspects of Their Jobs, by Departmental Location

Aspect of Trainer/Educator Job	Percent Indicating Need for More Information		
	All Departments (N=536*)	Nursing (N=262)	Education (N=82)
All respondents	100%	100%	100%
Evaluating inhouse training/education programs	63	63	70
Measuring training and nontraining costs	51	47	59
Evaluating packaged programs from outside sources	51	52	51
Creating tailored training materials	51	54	46
Assessing training/education needs	48	52	37
Setting measurable training objectives	48	49	44
Building learning principles into program designs	42	48	29
Combining elements of an educational program effectively	42	49	33
Achieving an effective instructional-methods mix	38	44	33

*Includes 31 respondents who did not indicate an informational need, and 192 in other departments, including administration, personnel, and staff development.

Table 18. Distribution of Respondents by Number of Aspects of Their Jobs About Which They Desired to Know More

Number of Aspects Designated	Number	Percent
All respondents	536	100
No aspect designated	31	6
One	23	4
Two	54	10
Three	103	19
Four	116	22
Five	66	12
Six	28	5
Seven	43	8
Eight	26	5
Nine	46	9

The degree of interest in learning more about measuring costs may be related to the respondents' degree of influence over acquiring funds. Trainers in education departments were more interested in learning more about measuring costs than those in other departments and, as has been noted, they also reported having more influence over acquiring funds.

Five or more aspects of the training job were designated by 39 percent of all respondents as areas of learning needs; nearly all of these 209 trainers (91 percent) expressed a need to learn more about evaluation of inhouse training programs. In fact, the proportion of those expressing needs in relation to each aspect was significantly greater than for any other group of respondents. The range was from 69 percent for measuring costs to 79 percent for creating materials and assessing needs.

Table 19. Percent of Respondents Indicating Desire to Know More About Specified Job Aspects, by Number of Aspects Designated

Aspect of Trainer/Educator Job	All Respondents Designating Specified Aspect (N=505)	Total Number of Aspects Designated			
		One or Two (N=77)	Three (N=103)	Four (N=116)	Five or More (N=209)
All respondents	100%	100%	100%	100%	100%
Evaluating inhouse training programs	67	30	58	58	91
Measuring training and nontraining costs	54	35	44	50	69
Evaluating packaged programs from outside sources	54	21	44	45	76
Creating tailored training materials	54	23	30	49	79
Assessing training education needs	51	17	29	41	79
Setting measurable training objectives	50	12	32	49	75
Building learning principles into program designs	45	10	23	41	70
Combining elements of an education program effectively	45	13	24	34	73
Achieving an effective instructional-methods mix	41	9	16	34	70

Among the five general categories initially listed, program implementation ranked last. The rankings of the three aspects included in this category—building learning principles into program designs, combining educational elements effectively, and achieving effective methods "mix"—were similar for the respondents as a whole; but respondents from nursing departments evidenced more needs for information about these aspects than did the whole group, and education department respondents evidenced fewer needs.

The contrast between the responses of education department trainers and of nursing department trainers is most striking in regard to building learning principles into program designs. Only 29 percent of the education department trainers, but 48 percent of the nursing department trainers, expressed their interest in learning more about this aspect of the trainers' job.

Institutional Training Needs

It has been noted that current programming was explored in relation to 12 areas of institutional training needs. Respondents were also asked to indicate whether, during the next two years, the needs of their hospitals in these areas would "probably increase," "remain unchanged," or "decrease" (Table 20, page 25).

Nearly four-fifths of all respondents predicted an increase in need for continuing education and supervisory development programs in their hospitals (Table 21, page 25). In six additional areas, increasing needs were predicted by more than 60 percent of all respondents. In order of rank, these areas were: patient education, orientation, interdepartmental relations and coordination, community health education, entry-level skills training, and upper management development. Very few respondents indicated that any needs would decrease in their hospitals, the largest proportion being the seven percent predicting a decrease in the need for entry-level skills training.

Here, again, departmental affiliation appears to have influenced responses. For nursing department trainers, continuing education headed the list (84 percent predicted increased need in this area); but for education and "other" department trainers supervisory development ranked first (82 percent and 81 percent respectively). The proportion predicting increased needs for continuing education, orientation programs, and entry-level skills training, was greater among nursing than among education or "other" department respondents, but the reverse was true for eight of the remaining specified items. Seventy-three percent of the education department respondents, but only 59 percent of the nursing department respondents and 67 percent of "other" respondents, forecast increasing needs for upper management development programs.

An equal proportion (79 percent) of both nursing and education department respondents expressed the view that patient education needs would be increasing in their hospitals; among both, this item ranked second.

As a whole, the respondents predicted that demand for their services would rise. It is important to bear in mind that each respondent's point of reference was the current situation in his own hospital. The information presented here reflects the situation in hospitals that were already committed to training activities, and may greatly understate the future training needs of the hospital field as a whole.

IMPLICATIONS OF SURVEY DATA

Survey respondents showed great interest in cooperation with educational institutions, and in shared training programs among hospitals. In fact, from a comparison of responses to this survey with data from the national survey of shared services previously mentioned, it would appear that hospitals employing professional trainers are more likely to share training programs than are other hospitals. One must remember that over three-quarters of the respondents to this survey are employed by hospitals having more than 200 beds. If hospitals with fewer than 200 beds (which comprise over 70 percent of the nation's hospitals) are much less likely than larger hospitals to employ professional trainers, these smaller hospitals are most in need of the educational expertise that could be provided to them through cooperative and shared programming. Investigation of the training needs of small hospitals, and demonstration or pilot programs of shared and cooperative services, would be valuable.

This survey focuses attention on the needs of hospital-based educators and trainers in terms of organizational support, outside resources, software, and their own continuing education. Trainers perceive their own most urgent continuing education need to be learning how to evaluate training programs carried out within their hospitals. They also need closely related instruction in how to measure training costs. They are amply supplied with educational hardware and are interested in using new educational methods and technology, but they need assistance in evaluating software from outside sources and in creating their own training materials. Nearly half of the respondents would like to learn more about assessing training needs. It also appears that trainers are unfamiliar with, or inexperienced in, the use of techniques employing objective data for reliable determination of needs.

Table 20. Distribution of Respondents by Their Expectation of Change in Training/Education Needs During Next Two Years

Training/Education Need	All Responses (N=536)	Expectation of Change in Need			
		Increase	No Change	Decrease	No Opinion
Continuing education	100%	79%	9%	—	12%
Supervisory development	100	79	9	1	11
Patient education	100	77	5	1	17
Orientation	100	73	18	3	6
Interdepartmental relations and coordination	100	70	7	1	22
Community health education	100	68	5	1	26
Entry-level skills training	100	65	17	7	11
Upper management development	100	64	13	1	22
Medical staff continuing education	100	41	8	—	51
Refresher training	100	40	19	5	36
Basic literacy training	100	17	20	3	60
English as second language	100	13	22	2	63

Table 21. Percent of Respondents Expecting Increased Training/Education Needs in Specified Areas During Next Two Years, by Departmental Location

Training/Education Need	All Departments (N=536)	Nursing (N=262)	Education (N=82)	Other* (N=192)
All respondents	100%	100%	100%	100%
Continuing education	79	84	76	72
Supervisory development	79	76	82	81
Patient education	77	79	79	76
Orientation	73	77	71	67
Interdepartmental relations and coordination	70	68	74	70
Community health education	68	68	72	73
Entry-level skills training	65	65	63	65
Upper management development	64	59	73	67
Medical staff continuing education	41	38	44	44
Refresher training	40	35	44	44
Basic literacy training	17	11	18	24
English as second language	13	11	13	16

*Includes respondents in administration, personnel, and staff development.

Hospitalwide training is evolving in many hospitals from long-established programs of nursing inservice training and nursing education. Half of the respondents were working in nursing service or nursing education. They need assistance to become expert directors of educational programming, in addition to being teachers of nursing knowledge and skills.

It appears that hospital-based trainers recognize a need for educational programs for the public served by hospitals, and they believe that patient and community health education, as well as continuing education for hospital personnel, should be part of their responsibilities. Although 77 percent of all respondents predicted increasing need for programs of patient education, only 30 percent reported ever having planned or conducted patient education programs. Similarly, although 68 percent predicted increasing need for programs of community health education, only 23 percent reported ever having planned or conducted such programs. The survey does not explain these gaps between the level of apparent need and the level of reported action, but it seems safe to suggest that trainers need assistance in planning and conducting programs of patient and community health education.

Substantial disparity between predicted needs and past performance also appears in the survey data in regard to continuing education for the medical staff (although this was generally outside the scope of the respondents' duties), programs for upper management and for first-level and second-level supervisory development, and programs to improve interdepartmental relations and coordination. Sixty-four percent of all respondents forecast increasing needs for upper management development programs, but only 36 percent had ever planned or conducted such programs. Seventy-nine percent predicted increasing needs for supervisory development; only 55 percent had planned or conducted such programs. Seventy percent expected increasing needs for programs to improve interdepartmental relations and coordination, but programs in this area had been planned or conducted by only 32 percent of the respondents. It appears that hospital-based trainers would also welcome assistance in planning and conducting programs to meet the needs of supervisors, department managers, and administrative personnel.

It is important to note that medical education—even continuing medical education —may be completely separate from the activities of these hospital-based trainers. Of all respondents, only 8 percent reported ever having planned or conducted continuing education for the medical staff; 51 percent reported "no opinion" as to future changes in demand for medical staff continuing education; and 52 percent reported that their hospitals had directors of medical education, but of these only one-third said that their activities and those of the directors of medical education were coordinated.

The survey findings suggest that trainers who are not specifically charged with hospitalwide programming may find it difficult to initiate programs to meet the perceived needs of personnel outside their own departments. It appears that trainers who are nurses may be most handicapped by this kind of situation. To meet needs adequately, it may be useful to institutionalize the training function as an office with hospitalwide responsibilities, crossing departmental lines.

3

The Hospitalwide Approach

The Hospital Continuing Education Project fostered what is still a rapidly growing national network of people concerned with the continuing education and training of hospital personnel. We assembled a cadre of program planners and material developers, a series of regional university centers for continuing education, and regional hospital organizations with education specialists. But the point of our work, and the work of all concerned, was not only to develop an educational delivery system, but to answer the question of how this system is to be completed in hospitals. Or, to put the question more pertinently, how can an individual hospital organize its resources, both internal and external, to fulfill its commitment to continuing education? Including continuing education within a coordinated hospitalwide program of education and training is the best answer.

What is meant by a hospitalwide program? How does it differ from training and educational activities of the past? The difference lies in this: hospitalwide education is directed by a central office with clearly defined accountability for education and training throughout the hospital. Responsibility for continuing education, for example, is lodged in the central office rather than within various departments, and the activities of the director of education cross departmental lines. A hospitalwide program may include (but need not be limited to) employee orientation, on-the-job training, inservice continuing education, supervisory and management development, and coordination of training to promote career mobility. Direction of a school of nursing and of professional internships and residencies may also be included; if not, their direction and planning should be coordinated with the planning of the department of education and training.

27

A serious commitment to hospitalwide continuing education, like the hospital's commitment to participation in preparatory education for medical and allied health careers, sensibly leads to some form of cooperation with other institutions. The director of a hospitalwide program is a link between the hospital and these outside resources— the developing network of continuing education directors in other hospitals, in state, regional and national hospital associations, in universities and other educational institutions, and in other professional associations and agencies interested in health care education.

The degree to which a hospital commits itself to providing hospitalwide education for its employees should be a matter for careful study and policy decision. Such a program represents a major commitment on the part of management—the board of trustees and the administration. It will require both human and financial resources. Besides staff costs and program fees, there will be overhead expenses for use of office and classroom space, materials and equipment to buy, travel to pay for, and, of course, costs incurred by releasing employees from duty. A hospital must ask itself: Is it all worth it? The answer to this question comes only from a searching examination of the institution and its objectives. What is the hospital trying to do? Why? What does it take to accomplish the job? To what extent may the hospital meet its goals through cooperation with other organizations?

INSTITUTING HOSPITALWIDE TRAINING AND EDUCATION

The administrative structure of a hospital may have to be reorganized to find a place for a central office of training and education, but where it will be located within a given hospital will depend on that hospital's educational policies, on the scope of activities to be directed, and, very likely, on the previous experience and resources of the hospital in regard to its training and educational functions. For example, an urban hospital with more than 1500 beds is developing a hospitalwide education program directed by an interdepartmental committee. The committee has begun by planning and implementing a hospitalwide orientation program. It is hoped that this committee will provide hospitalwide programs without disturbing the autonomous professions and departments in planning and conducting their own special educational programs.

In many hospitals today, it is the office of the director of nursing inservice education, with long experience in planning continuing nursing education, that is being expanded into a department of hospitalwide training; in others, the training and educational function is located as a service area within the personnel department. However, the most prevalent way to organize hospitalwide education today is to make it a separate department of the hospital.

As the responses to the survey of hospital-based trainers suggest, placing the director of education in a staff position helps him to secure the understanding and support of management. But regardless of where his office is located in the structure of the hospital, he also needs understanding and cooperation from all departments. Before implementing a hospitalwide program, he should make sure that its purposes and scope are fully explained to all hospital personnel, perhaps by conducting informational sessions for each shift, and he should continue to maintain effective communication with other department heads and with all those affected by training programs. It may also be useful to explain hospitalwide programming to interested community groups and news media.

Advantages of a Hospitalwide Program

On the basis of current evidence, administrators can expect that centralizing responsibility for education and training will yield the hospital distinct advantages. There have been reports from small hospitals as well as from large ones that hospitalwide direction and planning are more efficient means of using resources, of effecting innovations, of improving and upgrading employee performance, and of liaison with other institutions and agencies. Utilization of existing personnel is more efficient; it is easier to arrange for expert personnel to teach in departments other than their own when the need arises, or to participate in team teaching. Purchasing and utilization of educational materials and equipment are also more efficient and economical when centralized, and unnecessary duplication of purchases may be eliminated.

The hospital may be able to employ a director with training and experience in adult education. His role should be that of coordinator, consultant, and trainer of teachers, who will help hospital instructors to plan and evaluate their lessons and to use effective methods and materials. The director of a hospitalwide program is in a position to determine needs and recommend educational priorities from an overall point of view, and to evaluate programming by means of a consistent set of standards.

Career Mobility

With a hospitalwide program, the hospital's educational policies should be made to dovetail with its personnel policies. As the report of the National Advisory Commission on Health Manpower said in 1967, "simply making educational opportunities available will not assure their utilization . . . unless sufficient incentives are provided."

For years many occupations in the health care field have been dead-end. Health care employers, employees, unions, and educators now recognize that real payoffs result from establishing career mobility programs. By helping employees advance to jobs and incomes commensurate with their abilities and desires, hospitals should be able to alleviate shortages of skilled and semi-skilled manpower and to reduce employee turnover.

Employee participation in continuing education should be one of the criteria for salary increases and advancement or increased responsibility. Through the coordination of continuing education with planned career mobility programs, employees can be encouraged to upgrade their skills in order to be eligible for promotion. Hospitals' efforts in continuing education will be largely wasted unless they develop training systems geared to systems of promotion and to significant increases in wages and fringe benefits.[1]

---

1. A study of opinions expressed by aide trainees in a program conducted by the Hospital Research and Educational Trust, with funds from the U. S. Department of Labor, led to the following conclusions: (1) On-the-job training is a decisive factor in job satisfaction and can be of material assistance in maintaining a stable work force; (2) upgrading skills of trainees leads them to be optimistic about their immediate job satisfaction, educational potential, and, therefore, potential jobs; (3) counseling on realistic educational and career patterns could become part of the instructor's role, with good effect; and (4) specific programs should be planned to help workers attain realistic goals in education and work— for example, a nationwide program planned for training nursing aides to become licensed practical nurses.

Career mobility planning is useful for both professional and nonprofessional employees, for both skilled and unskilled workers. A career mobility program means, in the first place, the planning of sequences of jobs (career ladders) that have a common core of skills and knowledge, with each job in the sequence demanding progressively augmented knowledge and skills. Secondly, for each sequence of jobs, an educational sequence must be planned that will enable a qualified person to advance from one job to the next without unnecessarily duplicating previous training and experience.

The hospital will need to release employees for education and training during working time, and will need to offer counseling and whatever general or remedial education may be necessary for employees to take advantage of the specialized training programs. Because the hospital is committing itself to the principle of promotion from within, it will offer training in those job sequences in which there is reasonable assurance that participating employees will in fact be promoted to more highly skilled and better paid jobs after they complete the training. Educational sequences should be worked out in cooperation with educational institutions, and should include whatever employees may need to obtain certification, licensure, or accreditation.[2]

When the planning of hospitalwide training and education is coordinated with this kind of career mobility program, the director of education should develop a master career plan for each employee, with information about the experience, education, and skills required to advance. This plan, revised as necessary, would be available as a reference for the employee, his supervisor, the education and training department, and management. It would assist the director of education to identify training needs and to advise the administrator which programs and materials would merit expenditure of the hospital's time and dollars. A file of information about local and regional educational opportunities, including sources of financial aid, would also be useful in counseling employees.

To the other costs of educational programming, career mobility programming will add the costs of relieving employees for released-time training. To assess the net costs of this addition, the trainer or administrator will have to estimate whether, over a period of time, savings have resulted from reduced turnover of employees and better utilization of manpower.

One outstanding example of a career mobility program is that developed at the University of Chicago Hospitals and Clinics.[3] In operation in this program are three distinct career ladders—in nursing, in laboratory science, and in clerical work; general education classes; and remedial education in reading, English, and mathematics. All training for clerical careers, beginning with basic typing, is conducted within the hospital. There are classes to prepare ward secretaries and clinic coordinators for clerical work in the clinics and nursing units, and classes in medical terminology to prepare clerical workers for such jobs as physicians' secretaries and medical records transcribers. In the programs in nursing and laboratory careers, the hospital has worked out cooperative programming with educational institutions that give employees academic credit for programs previously taken in the hospital. As an example, the

---

2. See *Career Mobility: A Guide for Program Planning in Health Occupations* (Chicago: American Hospital Association, 1971).

3. Sally Holloway and Robert G. Holloway, Work-study career mobility program. *Hospitals, J.A.H.A.* 46: Aug. 16, 1972.

sequence in the laboratory career ladder begins with basic science, taught in the hospital, and continues with courses in a cooperating educational institution, leading first to certification as a laboratory assistant, then to an associate of arts degree as a medical laboratory technician, and finally to possible certification as a physician's assistant. An employee may leave the ladder for employment at any level or may continue upward, as he desires.

The director of education and training at the University of Chicago Hospitals and Clinics describes four guiding principles for career mobility programming:

1. Educational programs should focus on practical work activities and should be directly and specifically tied to mobility.

2. Programming for each individual employee should start at his level in the career mobility sequence.

3. Training at each level should add to the core of knowledge and skills that must be applied at the next level, to eliminate duplication of effort and loss of time, money, and motivation.

4. Educational components of the career mobility system inside and outside the hospital must be linked, so as to promote effective utilization of scarce teaching resources.

Educational Resources

Besides maintaining files of information for career planning, the office of education and training should also function as a clearinghouse of up-to-date information on educational materials and equipment. Hospital libraries, which in former years were limited to medical books and journals, are now evolving into information centers for all health care personnel and will be valuable resources for education and training programs. The director of education and the hospital librarian should cultivate a cooperative working relationship, taking a team approach to the problems of selecting, locating, and making available printed materials and audiovisual hardware and software.

One of the most useful functions of the director of a hospitalwide program is to identify and make use of resources outside the hospital—nearby health care institutions and agencies, local and state hospital associations, community colleges and universities, and federal agencies. It may be possible among hospitals to share programming, or the teaching services of technical specialists, or certain kinds of equipment. Hospital suppliers may be approached as sources of materials, films, and other aids, as well as for the services of lecturers to demonstrate and teach the operation of the equipment they manufacture. An aggressive search for inexpensive outside resources, for outside funding, or for sharing and other cooperative arrangements can make it possible for any hospital—however limited its educational budget—to provide a comprehensive educational program.

Budgeting

When education and training have become centralized as a distinct function, allocating particular resources to agreed-upon ends, then budgeting practices in force in other departments are applied to training. How funds are allocated to specific educational or training activities depends in part on the evolution of the training function in the hospital and the degree to which it has become established in a central office.

A number of interviews with directors of training in hospitals, business, industry, and university extension work have shown that there is a tendency for training directors to follow one of two general approaches to the formulation and implementation of budgets. For the sake of simplicity, these may be called the formal and informal approaches. The formal approach is characterized by a separate budget document under the operational control of the director of education. Under the informal approach, there is no such distinct document, and the director of education, by choice or by necessity, practices a strategy of influence and improvisation. In either case, budgeting for educational activities is generally based on a consideration of the estimated costs of meeting identified needs, rather than on trying to fix a rigid or arbitrary formula for expenditures.

In hospitals where the planning and conduct of training programs have not been centralized, but are departmental responsibilities, the informal approach to budgeting may be necessary. Instead of a formal budget under the control of the director of education, specific dollars are earmarked for educational programs within departmental budgets. Trainers practicing this approach stress that it may take time to build adequate departmental commitments to training activities. The director of education attempts to persuade department managers to incorporate continuing education objectives in their planning; keeps posted on the current status of their expenditures for training, and recommends specific additional programs for departments having the wherewithal; and identifies inexpensive resources and advises the departments on how to get the most for their educational dollars.

Formal budget documents containing specific categories of planned expenditures seldom come into being full blown. Directors of hospitalwide education and training may well take the initiative in pressing for the creation of budget documents, because they see certain advantages in controlling formal budgets. The existence of a budget may connote the commitment of the administration to training and education. Relative clarity may replace doubt as to the dollars authorized to cover expected costs. Decision-making authority (i.e., who has to check with whom in order to spend what) becomes defined.

Like the budgets of other organizational functions, training budgets usually do not require the expenditure of a stated number of dollars, nor do they represent inflexible or absolute limits on categories of expenditure. Some cost categories are unique to training and education. Training activities typically aim to serve the needs of personnel in other, "user" departments. For this reason, training directors often survey, more or less formally, the anticipated needs of these departments for particular programs for the forthcoming budget period. Almost 90 percent of the respondents to our survey of hospital-based trainers reported that they interviewed supervisors and department heads before making decisions on projected activities, and these interviews, together with informal conversations, were the methods they most frequently used to evaluate training needs. Employee questionnaires, performance evaluations, and records analysis were also used by over 60 percent, especially to determine needs for entry-level skills training and for continuing education.

Identified needs to be met generally provide the bases for estimating the costs of educational programming. Past experience, or the budget currently in force, serves as a guide to the cost of classes that have been conducted before, whether in the hospital or in a community college or university. The probable cost of a new program must be estimated by considering a number of factors, such as overhead, full-time or part-time salaries, the costs of releasing employees from duty, tuition charges, payments to faculty from outside the hospital, expenses for the purchase or rental of equipment, allowances for inflation of the costs of equipment to be purchased, costs to be charged back to the user departments, and so on.

It is useful to observe that the charge-back concept is gaining adherents among service-providing departments, such as training and personnel. Practice of the concept means prorating the costs of providing services among the user departments. Advantages are said to be the possibility of expanding activities and giving greater visibility to the service department; disadvantages are said to be the difficulty of prorating and the resistance of the user departments to service charges.

Current practice advocates that estimating the costs of meeting various needs be oriented to results; that is, the results to be expected from conducting specific activities and from expending particular sums should be estimated and compared. For instance, the estimated costs to be incurred may be compared for different numbers of classes to be taught, or for various kinds of skills to be acquired by estimated numbers of trainees. In the case of established programs, it may be considered whether savings would result from such changes as increased use of inhouse instructional talent or equipment, shared programming, or the use of new methods of teaching. Cost estimates thus take into account the work to be accomplished and the objectives to be met.

When it comes to gaining approval for a proposed educational budget, the crucial factors are the training office's reputation for performance, the quality of its relations with other departments and with administration, and its businesslike practices. Experienced training directors advise:

- Keep the budget simple and easily understood.

- Always be willing to discuss with department managers whether the results of training are worth the costs.

- Advocate your budgeted activities all during the year.

- Do not try to expand your budget too rapidly, or you will be viewed as greedy.

The director of education should be able to justify discrepancies between budgeted and actual expenditures, and any changes made from past budgets. Businesslike procedures, especially good record keeping, are essential.

Finally, attention should be paid to keeping budgets "on track." A system should be developed so that the director of education is notified periodically (once a month appears to be typical) of expenditures incurred and of the difference between budgeted and actual expenditures. For such information to be meaningful, the director needs the authority to make decisions within his budget, once it has been approved. Then he can, if necessary, make adjustments in spending rates or try to modify budgeted items.

Programs in Small Hospitals

Hospitalwide programming is proving to be as practicable for small hospitals as for large ones. In one very small rural hospital, the former director of nursing inservice education has become director of a hospitalwide program reaching employees, patients, and the community. Classes are repeated two or three times so that even part-time personnel find an opportunity to attend. A course on nutrition and special diets is taught by the head dietitian. Head nurses meet in a monthly seminar to examine problems involving their supervisory skills. The director of education has organized a library that includes a collection of do-it-yourself audio cassettes taped by persons who attend conferences and workshops and used by others who are unable to attend. She meets regularly, although informally, with a group of trainers from other small hospitals in the same part of the state.

Another small rural hospital recently employed its first director of hospitalwide training, who has a background in education. He is assisted by two part-time staff—a registered nurse and a secretary. He analyzes training needs through conversations and questionnaires and makes extensive use of packaged programs and training films. Members of the medical staff teach monthly classes on such topics as coronary care, intensive care, and athletic and farm injuries. The state university conducted an eight-week course in management and supervisory skills at the hospital with the participation of other local health care facilities. This hospital is investigating the possibility of forming an educational consortium with other institutions.

SHARING EDUCATIONAL SERVICES

"Hospitalwide" need not mean entirely supported by and limited to a single institution. Entering into an agreement to share educational services with one or more other hospitals is a form of cooperation which many hospitals recently have found advantageous (including more than half of those represented in the survey of hospital-based trainers), and in which many more are interested. The variety of possible sharing arrangements appears to be nearly unlimited. Some groups of hospitals that share educational services do so through informal agreements; others through formal contracts, or by setting up separate corporations. Still others share services through organizations to which they are related. Broadly speaking, there are at least four ways in which hospitals have been organizing shared services:

1. In the least formal arrangement, members of the group may refer their employees (for example, blood bank technicians) for training at one member hospital that maintains and controls a specific service.

2. A group of hospitals may arrange for and control the quality of a service that each individual institution purchases directly. For example, a group of hospitals may ask a community college to provide a supervisory training course. The curriculum will be planned jointly by the group and the college, but each

hospital will select the employees who are to attend and will pay their tuition directly to the college.

3. Educational services may be sponsored by professional associations; local hospital councils; state or regional hospital associations; religious orders; investor-owned chains; city, county, or state specialty organizations, such as purchasing groups; or regional planning agencies.

4. A group of institutions may organize a consortium to sponsor educational services. Components of a consortium may include one or more hospitals, health centers, extended care facilities, educational institutions or systems, planning agencies, or metropolitan or state hospital associations.

Consortium Arrangements

The consortium arrangement is very flexible. Through its director, the consortium may plan, conduct, and evaluate comprehensive educational programming, or it may provide only one specific kind of technical training to certain personnel from a number of hospitals. For example, a state university and five large teaching hospitals in a metropolitan area have formed a consortium for the purpose of developing and broadcasting closed-circuit color television programs for inservice training of hospital personnel, for continuing medical education, and for patient education. The university serves as the coordinating agency. Elsewhere, a state university with schools of medicine and nursing has joined a consortium of two investor-owned and two non-profit hospitals in a rural area. One of the hospitals, a city-owned institution that acts as the coordinating agency, participates in medical education and operates a hospital-wide program, including on-the-job training and continuing education, staff development, patient and public education, and an audiovisual aids library and production facility. Although in the past these institutions shared resources informally, the consortium arrangement has improved coordination of programming and has reduced unit costs.

By pooling resources, many rural hospitals have found it possible to obtain the services of an experienced professional educator who can direct inservice and continuing education and can act as liaison with educational institutions and government agencies. Three small rural hospitals in a southern state have realized just these advantages from their informal consortium. A large urban hospital in another predominantly rural state in the Southwest leads a consortium including four smaller hospitals, which has an outreach program offering educational planning and program implementation at a nominal charge for hospitals throughout the state. In the Midwest, a consortium of six hospitals in a farming area, ranging in size from fewer than 30 to more than 300 beds, has employed an experienced coordinator to assist administrative staff and supervisory personnel in each hospital in developing skills for designing, conducting, and evaluating inservice and continuing education. Another midwestern consortium of four urban hospitals is extending its hospitalwide programming to rural hospitals in a 13-county area, and finds the consortium arrangement an efficient means of coordinating and channeling the resources of state universities, local community colleges, and community agencies.

An educational consortium may be formally organized as a corporation, with a board of directors as the coordinating agency. For example, one consortium of four rural and urban hospitals and a community college is directed by a board of representatives from the county medical society, health planning agencies, and consumer groups, together with the head of the medical staff and the chairman of the board of directors from each of the member hospitals.

Any one of the component organizations may serve as the coordinating or lead agency for a consortium. Two recently formed consortiums are led by community colleges. A community college on the West Coast has organized a consortium of eight urban and suburban hospitals in its district in order to provide an effective, economical, and coordinated program with classes at the hospitals and on both of its campuses. Formerly, each hospital had to approach the college separately and use its services as best it could. A midwestern vocational-technical college with experience in six areas of health care education is directing a consortium of four medium-sized urban hospitals, and is integrating their existing educational programs with the program of the college in order to develop, conduct, and evaluate continuing education for the personnel of all the hospitals. This college has been able to secure partial state and federal funding. The extension division of a midwestern university is the lead agency of a consortium of very small rural hospitals and nursing homes, organizing training activities within or among institutions in response to needs analyses carried out under university direction. A state hospital association is the coordinating agency of another consortium of 10 suburban hospitals, a state college, and a technical school, which plans cooperative training to assist department heads, supervisors, and others to conduct their own programs for specialized groups within their hospitals.

National Survey of Shared Services

In 1971, a survey was made of shared continuing education and inservice training programs in short-term community hospitals in the United States; this was part of the national study of shared services, conducted by the Health Services Research Center, referred to in the previous chapter. The study surveyed a large sample of hospitals to find out which services hospitals were sharing, their satisfaction with those arrangements, and their interest in sharing other services (Table 22).

Relatively few of the hospitals surveyed reported sharing educational services, but a great many reported interest in joining with other hospitals to share these services in the future. The majority of sharing arrangements for continuing education and inservice training were satisfactory, although the number of programs apparently not found satisfactory raises the question of why they did not meet expectations.

A comparison of the survey results for New York state with those of a similar survey made there 14 months earlier shows a remarkable proliferation in implementation of and interest in shared programs during that period.

Evaluation of Shared Services

For the field of health care education in general, it seems that shared services may (1) reduce unnecessary and costly duplication of programs; (2) improve the communication of educational information among hospitals; (3) generate significant data

Table 22. Sharing of Continuing Education/Inservice Training Programs: Satisfaction with Shared Programs, Capability of Expansion to Other Hospitals, and Interest of Nonsharing Hospitals in Such Programs*

Category of Participants in Education/Training Program	Hospitals Sharing Specified Program				Number of Nonsharing Hospitals Interested in Sharing Program
	Number Sharing Program	Percent of All Responding to Survey	Number Satisfied With Program	Number That Could Expand Program to Others	
Clerical	151	3.2	99	84	524
Dietary	308	6.5	185	122	582
Housekeeping	184	3.9	116	101	556
Maintenance	161	3.4	91	94	565
Medical records	320	6.8	205	110	594
Nursing, general	538	11.4	332	176	681
Nursing, I.C.U.	701	14.8	452	217	685
Physicians' continuing education	699	14.8	447	219	654
Supervisory/management ..	421	8.9	243	150	662
Ward clerks	122	2.6	68	80	512

*These data are excerpted from the national survey of shared services conducted in July 1971 by the Health Services Research Center of the Hospital Research and Educational Trust and Northwestern University, in cooperation with the Bureau of Research Services of the American Hospital Association.

for forecasting manpower and training needs; and (4) facilitate manpower mobility among institutions.

But what about the individual hospital? Should most hospitals try sharing educational services? What makes a shared service successful? To seek answers to such questions, the Hospital Research and Educational Trust carried out an evaluation of a year's activities of one shared program—the Health Careers Training Program of Brooklyn, New York. This program was created in 1969 by six hospitals. A full-time director administered the program, and participating hospitals released employees for training during working hours and paid nominal rental fees for equipment. The shared training program was found to be practicable and valuable for the hospitals in the circumstances existing when they undertook it. The evaluation report of the Trust concluded that for shared training to be successful the following conditions are necessary:

1. *Commitment of hospital executives.* Hospital administrators must give firm support to the program in terms of financing, release of personnel for training, and personal involvement in the program. Responsibility for planning must be assumed by executives in the administrative and personnel departments of the participating hospitals, rather than by the central administrative agency or by lower-level management.

2. *Detailed planning and evaluation.* The role of the central administrative agency and its relationship with participating hospitals must be clearly defined. As a first step, training needs and objectives must be determined by the participating hospitals with assistance from the central agency. Needs and objectives should frequently be reexamined and redefined. Shared services must be integrated

with the training programs already existing within the participating hospitals. A continuing effort must be made to evaluate results against predetermined objectives in order to improve the program.

3. *Communication.* Continuing, effective communication must be maintained between the central agency and the participating hospitals. Close coordination must be maintained among the hospitals. Department heads and supervisors must be made fully aware of all phases of the shared program and of any changes made in it, to ensure their support and cooperation.

By sharing services, individual hospitals may augment and enrich the educational opportunities they can provide their employees. They may have the benefit of experienced leadership, expert faculty, and equipment and materials that they could not otherwise obtain or afford. For smaller hospitals with the motivation to develop hospitalwide training, a pooling of resources with one or more other health care institutions in the same area—perhaps coupled with the assistance of a community college or a state university—can help to bring about a program that will be of service to the entire region. On the other hand, not only is it difficult to create an organizational structure in which autonomous individual hospitals will have enough confidence to relinquish some control over decision making but also it is hard to maintain cooperation among these hospitals and their personnel.

IMPLEMENTING HOSPITALWIDE PROGRAMMING

Whether to share services, or to work out a cooperative program with a community college or university, is one of many decisions to be made when a hospital sets up hospitalwide programming. Hospitals vary in size, environment, scope and volume of services, and proximity to educational institutions and to other health care facilities. Successful development of hospitalwide programs in different situations will require different strategies.

A look at hospitals that have recently begun hospitalwide training programs yields many examples of adaptation to different specific problems. A large university hospital is under pressure from unions to set up a career ladder system with improved skills training. A rapidly expanding urban hospital is faced with a proliferation of specialty services and a drastic increase in numbers of personnel. On the other hand, a small rural hospital is hard-pressed to locate experienced manpower, and is trying to develop a modular program in which only one or a few employees can be trained at a time, without much interruption of work schedules. A city hospital that also recruits from an untrained labor force—except that these employees are members of minority groups whose general educational background is poor—is preparing its supervisory staff to become skilled trainers and is emphasizing career development. Another university hospital is planning cooperative training programs with the university school of allied health professions. In all these situations at least one factor is common: to a great extent, each director of education and his staff has had to pioneer. There are no widely tested or accepted guidelines for organizing hospitalwide programming, or for expanding existing departmental programs into hospitalwide ones.

Administrators and staff members who have been charged with developing hospital-wide educational programs have been asking for assistance in answering questions such as these:

1. How can institutional goals and policies be translated into educational objectives?

2. What should be the scope of a hospitalwide program in a given hospital? If the direction of all educational activities of the hospital—including medical internships and residencies, the hospital school of nursing, and preparatory education for allied health occupations—is not to be centralized, how are the medical and nonmedical programs to be coordinated?

3. What form should the educational and training function be given, and where should it be located in the organizational structure of the hospital?

4. What guidelines may be applied in expanding the educational and training function from activities centered in departments to a central program? What will be the relationship of the director of the hospitalwide program to technical instructors in other departments?

5. What will be the relationship of the office of hospitalwide education to outside agencies, voluntary organizations, and educational institutions that supply educational and training services? To other hospitals?

6. Are there guidelines for sharing educational services?[4] How may shared services be evaluated?

7. How can the hospitalwide educational program be coordinated with other programs—such as management engineering—to increase efficiency and quality in the delivery of health care?

Who will answer these questions? There is an urgent need to develop, test, and document a variety of hospitalwide educational and training programs, with the purpose of identifying models that can be replicated by other hospitals in similar circumstances.[5]

Model Programs

Two categories of model programs are needed: those for the single hospital and those for the consortium or group of institutions and agencies entering into a shared educational service project. Model programs should demonstrate how hospitalwide education and training can be organized, administered, and integrated into the management process in single hospitals, under three sets of circumstances:

1. Models for hospitalwide programs in single hospitals without preservice schools or clinical affiliations

---

4. Guidelines for shared educational programs are in preparation by the Hospital Research and Educational Trust. They will deal with identifying an institution's need for shared educational service programs, analyzing possible alternatives, and planning for implementation.

5. The Hospital Research and Educational Trust is the principal participant in a project assisted by the W. K. Kellogg Foundation, initiated in September 1972, to study hospitalwide education and training at 33 demonstration sites representing hospitals and consortiums of hospitals with educational institutions and other agencies.

2. Models for hospitalwide programs in single hospitals with preservice allied health education, on-the-job training, and continuing education under coordinated direction

3. Models for hospitalwide programs in single hospitals with medical internships and residencies, as well as preservice education, on-the-job training, and continuing education programs under coordinated direction

Particular attention must be paid to the training problems and needs of small hospitals. This is still a nation of predominantly small hospitals. Approximately 60 percent of the short-term general and special hospitals have 100 beds or less, and about 35 percent have fewer than 50 beds. Nevertheless, hospital literature contains little data on the operating characteristics of small hospitals to indicate their special needs or to justify the assumption that their educational needs are in fact distinct. A number of questions about training in small hospitals come immediately to mind:

1. Which persons are responsible for training? How have they been prepared for their instructional roles?

2. What training methods are employed? Why were these methods chosen in preference to others? How effective are these methods?

3. To what extent are small hospitals able to meet their training needs? What outside educational resources do they use?

4. What factors make it possible for some small hospitals to carry out active programs of training and education, while others are able to do little?

A variety of model programs for consortium relationships should also be developed to demonstrate how different combinations of institutions may work together to do an effective job of education and training. For health care facilities, educational institutions, and associations that are interested in shared programming, data are needed on different methods of determining the financial obligations of the members of consortiums, on the relative advantages of formal and informal organization, on methods of dealing with common educational needs of members and with individual needs, and on methods of competing for and obtaining outside resources.

Hospitals are on the threshold of expanding hospitalwide education and training programs. The few examples observed to date and the models presently being developed give cause for optimism. Other hospitals should watch these developments closely and be encouraged to undertake experimentation.

4

Cooperative Programs With Educational Institutions

From vocational schools to universities, educational institutions can make as great a contribution to continuing education in health care as they do to preservice education. Four-fifths of the trainers responding to the national survey reported that their hospitals are now engaged in one or more kinds of cooperative training programs with educational institutions, especially vocational-technical schools, community colleges, and universities.

WORKING WITH COMMUNITY COLLEGES

Community colleges constitute the fastest growing segment of American higher education. Including these colleges in cooperative or shared service arrangements is especially attractive, because they have two significant advantages for hospital continuing education: their accessibility to employed adults who cannot leave daily work to attend classes beyond commuting distance, and their flexibility in tailoring programs to local needs. It is the responsibility of the hospital, or hospital association, and its director of education to initiate a working relationship with the community college.

When a hospital and a college arrange a cooperative educational program for hospital personnel, and especially when a college is invited to conduct classes on the hospital premises, it is very important to spell out clearly the obligations of the hospital, the college, and the participating employees, and to make sure that all parties understand them. An explicit agreement should cover liability, security policies, schedules, and the use of classrooms and other hospital facilities and equipment. The hospital director of education should be responsible for communicating to prospective students the conditions of attendance, registration procedures, and fees. The hospital will have to decide whether or not to schedule classes as part of the employees' working time and whether to pay all or part of their fees. The hospital should offer every possible assistance to the cooperating college and its faculty.

Universities, Community Colleges, and Hospitals

All avenues of cooperation with community colleges should be of paramount interest to directors of education in hospitals and hospital associations. One interesting possibility is to add a third partner—a university—to the combination of hospital and community college. The supervisory training program of the Office of Continuing Hospital and Health Care Education at the University of Minnesota extends continuing education opportunities to full-time hospital employees in several states through community colleges.[1] This program suggests an alternative to training that requires periods of residence on a university campus.

The need to make supervisory training accessible to hospital personnel in their own communities was ranked first in a survey of the educational needs of hospitals in the Upper Midwest conducted in 1965 by the Office of Continuing Hospital and Health Care Education, which was one of the Hospital Continuing Education Project's university centers. With the cooperation of the state hospital associations in the region, the center asked five colleges[2] to participate in a supervisory training program. The relationship between the colleges and the University of Minnesota, and their mutual obligations, were stipulated in formal agreements, signed by representatives of each college and the university administration. Because these unique cooperative relationships between a large state university and community colleges were responsible for the success of the Minnesota supervisory training program (which was later extended to other communities and other states), a summary of the contractual arrangements might be of interest.

Each college agreed to offer a course in supervisory training for full-time employees of hospitals in their communities or within commuting distance, and to appoint a faculty coordinator, who was free to invite qualified practitioners to assist him in teaching. The coordinators also worked with advisory committees appointed by the state hospital associations, which included the administrators of local hospitals and hospital association executives.

The university, through the center, provided modest financial support. The center sponsored a workshop on curriculum for the faculty coordinators before the opening of courses, and another on evaluation at their close. The center also provided a curriculum topic outline, a bibliography, reference materials, and sample teaching materials and tests. The syllabus for each course, however, was designed at each college by the faculty coordinator and his advisory committee to meet the needs of their students and to take advantage of the know-how of local faculty members,

---

1. This program is described in detail in *Supervisory Training: The University, The Community College, and The Hospital* (Chicago: Hospital Research and Educational Trust, 1971).
2. The five colleges are Bismarck Junior College, Bismarck, N. Dak.; Dakota Wesleyan University, Mitchell, S. Dak.; Marshalltown Community College, Marshalltown, Iowa; United College (now the University of Winnipeg), Winnipeg, Man., Canada; and Willmar State Junior College, Willmar, Minn.

experts from business and industry, and health care executives.

The decentralized approach of this model for university-community college-hospital programming has made it possible for the University of Minnesota to make a needed contribution to training in widely separated hospitals in an area including 10 states and the province of Manitoba.

WORKING WITH UNIVERSITY CENTERS

As the Minnesota program demonstrates, the development of regional university centers can be a key factor in expanding and improving continuing education opportunities for hospital personnel. The concept of regionalization is similarly being tried in medical and allied health education with the development of area health education centers relating to a university medical center, and for much the same reason: the contribution that backup university resources can make toward improving the quality of education. The unique advantages of the university lie in scholarly research and educational expertise, and hospitals need to draw upon these resources to improve training and educational methods and to bridge the gap between today's most advanced health care knowledge and its application in actual patient care.

Although the seven regional university centers of the Hospital Continuing Education Project were located in universities with graduate programs in hospital administration, which obviously had special resources, there is no reason why hospitals cannot work just as effectively with other universities to develop local or regional programs. Every university that has faculty oriented to health care delivery and a desire to contribute to continuing education in the field of health care should be encouraged to do so. University centers throughout the United States could stimulate and coordinate creative programming for their service regions.

Guidelines for Organizing Centers

In organizing a center, the first consideration must be the values and resources of the university, rather than hospitals' specific needs. There can be no single model, because universities differ in so many factors affecting planning. For example, there is an historic difference between public and private institutions with regard to their support of continuing education. A private university without a history of extension education or direct public service commitments may find it difficult to allocate financial support or to offer academic credit for continuing education courses. Among pertinent factors to consider are the university's previous experience in continuing education; its degree of commitment to community service; its previous relationships with hospitals, with local and regional health care associations, and with other educational institutions; its fields of research and expert knowledge that can be shared with continuing education students and with hospital educators; and the interest of its faculty members.

The location of the center within the university structure should be such that it will facilitate productive relationships with faculty in health administration programs, in extension programs, in industrial relations, or in any department of the university with pertinent resources.

Productive relationships with university faculties depend to a great extent on staff work by the center coordinators, who should be conversant with the structure and aims of the university and of hospitals and health care associations. The coordinators may work with formal advisory committees of faculty members and of association representatives, as well as through informal contacts with these groups and others. Sally Knapp, Ed.D., coordinator of the center at Columbia University, expressed the qualifications of an ideal coordinator: "The coordinator should be an able administrator; someone adept politically, who can get support from the university structure; someone with ability in behavioral science, who can stimulate his students; someone who knows what constitutes good teaching, and can find and use talented staff and faculty. The university must give the coordinator a certain amount of freedom if he is to be creative and to develop a program that meets real needs."

The first step in planning the center's program is to delineate the center's service region. How broad a geographical region can a university serve in this way? The answer to this question must not be arbitrary, because existing relationships will have to form the basis for the kind of cooperation among hospitals, associations, and educational institutions that will enable hospital personnel to take advantage of what the center has to offer. The scope of the service region must be determined by the resources of the center and by the extent of existing ties between the university and the educational and health care institutions in surrounding communities or states.

To determine hospitals' educational needs, it would be well to invite directors of education or other representatives of hospital and professional associations in the region to form an advisory committee. This committee also could assist with coordination of programming. Reliable surveys of needs should precede specific program development, and would then be available as data for later evaluation.

Finding sufficient financing to develop effective learning experiences is a long-range problem for universities and other institutions offering continuing education. Most students may come from hospitals with limited funds for tuition. Registration fees for on-campus courses may cover direct expenses for planning, promotion, materials, and faculty compensation; but there are still the initial costs of organizing the center and developing a program, and such long-range costs as office expenses and the operating funds that are required for needs determination, interagency cooperation, curriculum and materials development, educational research, and evaluation studies. In the past, federal agencies, university general funds, and hospital and professional associations have subsidized such programs. New sources of funds must be identified for the future, or more of the burden will have to be shared by the health care institutions that utilize the programs.

To be successful, the center must have wholehearted support from the university administration and faculty. Several coordinators from the Hospital Continuing Education Project centers reported that developing, revising, and conducting programs of university caliber take more time and effort than the faculty had anticipated. Adult education is not a condensed version of graduate or undergraduate education but requires attention to the motivation and needs of adult, employed students. Teaching only by lectures and assigned reading is less effective than using small workshops, role playing, computer games, in-basket exercises, and other methods involving active student participation.

According to Dr. Knapp, "The key to planning a work load for continuing education students is to put enough variety in it to avoid fatigue. Daily preparation must be stimulated by learning activities. In the Columbia course in management for hospital department heads and assistant administrators, when a problem-solving project was organized around an actual hospital situation, small groups of students met in the evening, of their own accord, to find solutions in preparation for the next day's class. Continuing education students are prepared to work, but if you stimulate evening assignments, rather than superimpose them, you get better results." For classes that are conducted on campus, it is important to have faculty who take a real interest in the program and are available for informal association with students.

Programming for University Centers

There are two basic approaches to long-range program planning for the university continuing education center. One approach is for the university to act as a "facilitator," to stimulate and assist other institutions and professional associations to develop their own educational programs. The center may make university resources and skills available directly to training and education officers in hospitals and hospital associations, or indirectly through colleges and local school districts or as a member of a consortium or other sharing arrangement. The University of Minnesota adopted this approach to a greater extent than any of the other centers in the Hospital Continuing Education Project. The other approach is to plan, promote, and conduct a program of continuing education, on or off campus, directly under university auspices. These two approaches are by no means exclusive, but each has different implications for staffing, financing, and selecting the categories of hospital personnel to be reached.

Programs conducted directly by the university should be those that the university is best equipped to offer and that are not otherwise available in the region. In addition to their graduate programs in hospital administration, most universities participating in the Hospital Continuing Education Project were already offering some continuing education courses in health care management, generally consisting of short institutes on specific topics. The project gave impetus to the planning of longer programs that offered hospital administrators, department managers, and supervisory personnel more thorough study and learning experiences. The experience of the project suggests that short institutes and conferences on topics of immediate interest may be suitably and successfully offered to hospital personnel by metropolitan, state, and regional hospital associations, but that longer, in-depth courses are more appropriate for the university.

Even in a traditional "program conductor" role, a center can experiment with a variety of approaches to programming, as the activities of the project centers illustrate. Because they were closely related to graduate schools of hospital administration, many of their activities focused on management development. The center at Columbia University, for example, had a three-fold program. One aspect was offering courses: a year-long course in management development for hospital administrators, an adaptation of this for department heads and assistant administrators, and a variety of short courses. Second, at the request of state hospital associations, the center cosponsored programs or provided consultation. The third aspect was continuing education for the state association executives, who asked for programs related to their own careers and personal development.

The Western Center for Continuing Education in Hospital and Related Health

Institutions, at the University of California, used the university campus as a "neutral meeting ground" or forum, where the center could bring together professional and administrative health care personnel in working conferences. Because of the large number of nursing homes in the state, the center adopted as one of its goals improving the coordination of the health professions relating to patient care, both in hospitals and nursing homes. At one time or another, participants in the working conferences included hospital and nursing home administrators, members of voluntary and governmental agencies, physicians, nurses, dietitians, medical social workers, pharmacists, and therapists. The center hoped that the conferences might set a pattern for working relationships within individual institutions.

An innovative summer series of five-day institutes under the title, "Life-long Learning," was inaugurated by the center at the University of Michigan, with somewhat disappointing but instructive results. The center's original plan was to offer a limited number of intensive institutes every summer and revise them annually, so that students would be able to return to the campus for one or two weeks every summer and not encounter repetition of subject matter. The institutes were open to experienced hospital administrators and executives of planning and prepayment agencies throughout the United States, and were based on current research by members of the university faculty. Topics included "Planning Health Services," "Measuring Hospital Performance," "Unit Management," and "Reimbursement." Although the institutes attracted capacity enrollment and were very favorably evaluated the first time they were offered, the following year, when they were repeated, attendance dropped sharply. It appeared that the research orientation and level of difficulty of some subjects had a limited appeal to prospective students, and therefore a limited audience, and perhaps lacked immediate relevance for most administrators. In addition, the necessity to take time from work and the expenses of tuition and living costs were important constraints. Although faculty were interested in presenting the results of their research, they were less interested in repeating institutes, especially during the summer. Thus, the center was forced to conclude that its "Life-long Learning" format was not practical as a long-range continuing education program for administrators.

The centers at Duke University and St. Louis University both organized courses for hospital administrators and assistant administrators based on their master's degree programs. The St. Louis University summer program enrolls 30 new students annually for a three-summer sequence of classes. The one-year Hospital Administrators Management Improvement Program at Duke University was designed for the executive officers of hospitals in North Carolina and South Carolina, where there are large numbers of small community hospitals. A group of 24 students attends an initial one-week session of classes at the university in September and two-day meetings in each of the following 11 months.

RESIDENTIAL–HOME-STUDY PROGRAMS FOR ADMINISTRATORS

It is very likely that administrators of small hospitals have been promoted to their positions without formal preparation for top-level management, because most hospitals are not administered by alumni of university programs in hospital administration.

Program graduates often find better prospects for advancement by accepting positions as assistant administrators in large hospitals than by becoming administrators of hospitals with fewer than 100 beds. Many program graduates also are attracted by opportunities in government, prepayment plans, or planning agencies. The Hospital Continuing Education Project was especially concerned with finding ways to use university resources to meet the development needs of administrators of small hospitals without disrupting their work schedules. This concern led the project staff to experiment with a format for programming that has become known as the "residential–home-study" course.

Several universities were encouraged to conduct a solid two-week program of on-campus study, followed by 11 months of individualized study back home (not to be tainted by calling it a "correspondence course," which would have been an inaccurate description), and then two final weeks of study on campus designed to be relevant to what had happened to the students during the home-study period. These courses were not recommended for preservice training or as substitutes for graduate degree programs; rather, enrollment was limited to chief administrators of hospitals (and in some cases, nursing homes) who had had at least one year or more of experience in their positions, but no formal education in health care administration. If academic credit could be given by the universities, so much the better. The curriculums emphasized the application of up-to-date theory and techniques to students' current management problems.

A good example of a residential–home-study program is that offered by the Center for Health Services Continuing Education at the University of Alabama. The heart of the course is the development of a simulation model of a typical hospital, including a complete budget, financial statement, and personnel profile and problems; all subjects relate to this model. On the campus, lectures are supplemented by a variety of audio-visual materials, and students engage in role playing, simulation exercises, administrative in-basket exercises, and seminars. During the home-study period, a student works at monthly lessons comprised of readings, case studies, and questions on topics closely related to the daily operation of his own hospital. Completed lessons are reviewed by university faculty and then forwarded to the student's preceptor, an experienced practicing administrator in a nearby hospital, who meets regularly with the student to discuss practical aspects of the lessons. Although begun as a noncredit course, the Alabama residential–home-study program now offers either baccalaureate or college credit to the 50 students who enroll annually.

The Office of Continuing Hospital and Health Care Education at the University of Minnesota has worked out an interesting variation of the residential–home-study format, the Independent Study Program, for top-level hospital administrators in its service area: Iowa, Kansas, Manitoba, Minnesota, Missouri, Montana, Nebraska, North Dakota, South Dakota, and Wisconsin. This is a three-year sequence of courses planned to develop the student's capacity for self-directed learning. Students may earn academic credit through the extension division of the university. Each year's course contains all or most of these components: a residential session on campus at the beginning and end of each course; seminar sessions at sites throughout the Upper Midwest; monthly home-study unit lessons, each covering a specific topic; and preceptor-student dialogues. There also is a training program for the administrators who serve as preceptors. Each preceptor meets monthly with a group of students, and students present and criticize formal papers at periodic regional seminars that combine at least two preceptorial groups.

A significant feature of this program is the extensive collection of study materials prepared at the university and made available only to enrolled students. Handbooks explain study techniques. Unit lessons, mailed monthly to first-year and second-year students, include a statement of objectives, copies of required readings, references to optional reading, and a list of performance assignments such as written papers, case studies, or problem definitions. Third-year students receive a packet of study materials for each topic covered.

The first-year course is concerned with the internal management and organization of the hospital; the second year, with relationships among the various departments and functional groups within the hospital, including the board of trustees and medical staff; the third year, with external forces affecting the delivery of health care. Through a multimethod approach, students are given increasing responsibility for the content and process of learning, leading in the final year to an independent demonstration or research project supported by a scholarly paper. The third-year course is open to those who have successfully completed the second year, to those with a master's degree in hospital administration, and to executives of health care agencies and organizations. Students may repeat the third year periodically to study different topics.

Correspondence Education

The value of combining home study with contacts on the campus and with the preceptors was stressed in the results of a study of correspondence education undertaken by the Hospital Continuing Education Project concurrently with its establishment of the residential–home-study programs. Research into the use and potential of correspondence instruction as a method of continuing education among all categories of hospital employees was carried out for the project by Pennsylvania State University.[3] The study found that correspondence instruction has proved to be an effective teaching and learning method in many fields, but that hospitals made little use of it, and, in fact, that relatively few hospitals were aware of the availability of suitable correspondence courses.

Correspondence education was not highly regarded by respondents, although students and educators who had had experience with it were more favorably inclined toward its use than those who had not. Hospital administrators were reluctant to use correspondence instruction because of what they perceived to be great difficulty in maintaining employees' motivation to complete the courses. In the opinion of a panel of 25 experts on correspondence instruction who were consulted in the study, its effectiveness depends on the degree to which courses are structured to reinforce motivation and to achieve communication between students and instructors. The panel recommended the use of audiovisual media, including television; programmed instruction; personal assistance from hospital staff members; and the combination of on-campus instruction with correspondence study.

---

3. For a summary and analysis of this research, including recommendations, see *Correspondence Education and the Hospital* (Chicago: Hospital Research and Educational Trust, 1969).

Problems in Using the Residential–Home-Study Format

Although the residential–home-study format has been welcomed by administrators, it makes considerable demands on the resources and ingenuity of university staff. Enrollment must be limited according to the number of faculty and staff available. Finding qualified preceptors is difficult, and some programs have substituted group seminars or combined preceptorial conferences with seminars, benefiting from the added input of many points of view. Developing, revising, and administering correspondence lessons, in addition to preparing on-campus sessions, are especially time-consuming and expensive.

Representatives of the universities whose residential–home-study programs were funded through the Hospital Continuing Education Project expressed interest in the idea of organizing some kind of umbrella agency to coordinate and expand these programs, possibly with centralized administration of the home study lessons. Each of the programs funded through the project was autonomous in planning and administration. If universities could participate in a program under national auspices, more of them might become interested in offering this type of course. With the exception of public institutions with extension services, there has been great reluctance among universities to engage in any type of correspondence instruction. A central agency might be able to overcome the poor reputation of correspondence lessons by producing materials of high quality, in addition to reducing expenses and relieving the universities of the burden of home study administration.[4] However, a centralized program would probably require some common organization of curriculums by university faculties in order to accommodate the residential sessions to standardized correspondence materials.

In view of the rapidly changing range of presently available educational opportunities for hospital administrators, as well as the increasing use of such media as television and audio cassette recordings for long-distance education, it would seem wise to defer a major commitment to future expansion of residential–home-study programs for hospital administrators until a survey of the potential market for such an expansion has been completed.

The most attractive potential use of this format may well be to offer training in administrative skills to middle managers and department heads, including nursing service directors, who have been promoted to administrative positions from the technical ranks of health care professionals. The center for hospital continuing educa-

---

4. Many functions that might usefully be performed by a central agency for hospital-oriented correspondence instruction are suggested in the report, *Correspondence Education and the Hospital*. Among these are:

   1. Maintenance of a clearinghouse to file and disseminate information on correspondence courses applicable to the learning needs of hospital personnel.
   2. Assembly of a core group of specialists to promote the adaptation of existing courses, and to develop new courses in areas not covered.
   3. Promoting and conducting research leading to improved quality in correspondence courses.
   4. Encouraging hospitals to make greater use of correspondence instruction, and to develop policies for employees relating to financial support, time allowed for study, staff assistance, and benefits to be obtained by completion of courses.

tion at Columbia University had great success in adapting the format of its residential–home-study program for administrators to management development for assistant administrators and department managers. Similar programs have been introduced in Canada. After finding that not more than 10 percent of the nursing service directors in the Upper Midwest have had formal academic preparation in administration, the University of Minnesota center has recently established such a program for nursing service directors and patient care administrators.

PREPARING HOSPITAL EDUCATORS AND INSTRUCTORS

So far this chapter has described some experimental and some current university programs of hospital continuing education. I would like to propose another kind of activity, as yet untried. There is a severe shortage of persons who are skilled in planning, administering, and teaching in programs designed to improve the job performance of hospital personnel, and this shortage affects both on-the-job training and continuing education, in both hospital-based programs and those sponsored by hospital and professional associations. I would propose that universities in different regions of the United States provide training facilities to prepare hospital administrators and instructors for managing and teaching in hospital training and education programs.

Administrators need to know how to organize and support training efforts and how to create a climate within the hospital in which training can produce real changes and improvements. Directors of education and training need assistance in managing programs and in developing the teaching skills of other hospital instructors. Most training in hospitals, even those in which there is a director of education, is carried out by professionals—by department heads or supervisory personnel—who need assistance to become effective teachers. Introducing these instructors (who may be, for example, nursing supervisors or medical technologists) to current teaching methods and providing them with appropriate training materials are the principal steps in initiating new training and continuing education programs.

Instructor training centers should be organized on a regional basis at a number of universities and should pursue the following objectives:

1. To prepare administrators and directors of education to manage hospital-based education and training

2. To increase the number of skilled instructors in the hospital field

3. To determine the most effective methods of developing the teaching skills of content-oriented specialists

4. To disseminate their findings

These regional centers should be located in universities with proven records of success in extension and continuing education, and should be directed by experienced educators. To achieve the objectives, university hospitals and university departments of psychology, education, and continuing education should be closely linked. Effective curriculums would concentrate on giving hospital-based instructors experience with a variety of teaching and learning techniques. Advisory committees appointed by the universities could represent the needs of the region's hospitals and professional community.

This chapter has only begun to explore the ways in which universities can contribute to continuing education. Working in concert with hospital associations and professional organizations, universities can be a strong resource. Just as the roles of universities must be carefully spelled out, so must the roles of hospital associations. The next chapter defines the role of hospital organizations and their education directors.

5

Association Directors of Education

Bringing continuing education within the reach of every hospital worker will take the combined efforts of hospitals, of colleges and universities, and of hospital associations at all levels. Each has a distinctive contribution to make. National associations cannot and should not try to offer the kinds of services to individual hospitals that can be contributed by intermediate organizations at regional, state, or local levels.

By adopting the role of facilitator, university centers have been able to stimulate and improve regional and local educational opportunities for health care personnel, in addition to offering on-campus courses. Similarly, by setting up offices for directors of education who are responsible for developing programs, state and regional hospital associations have been able to offer many educational services to hospitals in addition to their customary institutes and short courses.

ROLES AND FUNCTIONS

Regional Hospital Association's Role

The only regional hospital association that was part of the Hospital Continuing Education Project's director of education program was the New England Hospital Assembly. The assembly had existed for almost fifty years as an organization of hospitals in six states. Its sole purpose was to offer continuing education for hospital personnel. Unlike some areas of the country where we tried, sometimes not very successfully, to create arbitrary "regions" for the purpose of the project, the New England Hospital Assembly area was already a compact region with social, economic, and, of course, educational ties, and with educational institutions easily reached from

53

all points. The question we asked was how to put those resources to work on a better-organized basis. What might be the distinctive contribution of a regional association to continuing education?

The New England Hospital Assembly had always relied on the energetic and dedicated labors of volunteers. With increasing demands being made on health manpower, and the importance of training in meeting those demands, the New Englanders decided that they wanted a full-time director of education. They reached this conclusion not without some anxiety on the part of the leadership that the existence of such a staff member might discourage the volunteer effort that had sustained the assembly for so long.

The direction taken by the assembly's educational programming since the appointment of a director of education has been largely influenced by the decision to locate his office at the New England Center for Continuing Education. The center had been established by the W. K. Kellogg Foundation at the University of New Hampshire, with the involvement of all six New England state universities. As Richard Allen, the assembly's director of education, explains it, there seemed to be an opportunity in New England to use the center to link the hospitals with its educational institutions. This was accomplished by a tripartite agreement between the New England Center and the New England Hospital Assembly, with the University of New Hampshire as fiscal agent. The agreement established an Office of Health Care Education as the element of the New England Center responsible for conducting all programs in health care continuing education. The assembly's director of education was named director of this office, reporting jointly to the center and to the assembly.

According to Allen, "We have developed a new focus in which both state and private educational institutions are equal partners and equal contributors in a total regional program. We are working on plans to promote mutual cooperation among vocational-technical institutes, community colleges, universities, and hospitals in developing health care education that meets real needs. Our intent is not to conduct all continuing education activities for New England, but to be a communications link. We would like to serve as an interface between the health industry and the knowledge industry."

Although the programming of the Office of Health Care Education has not been strictly confined to hospitals or to continuing education, educational programs have been primarily focused on hospitals. One aim has been to facilitate long-range planning to ensure the development of continuing education programs in all the community hospitals of New England. Programs have been conducted to "train the trainers" and to inform them of available resources. The director of education has expanded working relationships with the executives of the state hospital associations, providing counsel and support for specific programs, and locating state association programs that could be shared with other states. For example, the Office of Health Care Education agreed to bring to the attention of the entire region a Connecticut Hospital Association program on identifying and organizing feasible shared service arrangements among hospitals. The Office of Health Care Education also has secured the cooperation of four Regional Medical Programs and the New England Regional Commission in beginning regional planning for health care manpower and related education and training.

Members of the assembly continue to plan their traditional annual meeting, instructional conferences, and training institutes on a volunteer basis, with programming consultation and administrative services from the Office of Health Care Education. Richard Allen believes that the new directions taken by his office, rather than detracting from volunteer effort, have added a new dimension to the leadership role of the New England Hospital Assembly in health care education.

State and Local Hospital Associations' Roles

State and local hospital associations are in an excellent position to assess training needs, to assist hospitals to plan educational programs, and to tap the resources of professional societies, Regional Medical Programs, and educational institutions. In several state associations, the directors of education have been able to coordinate the work of these groups in relation to hospitals, as a few capsule descriptions of their activities during the Hospital Continuing Education Project will illustrate.

For example, in 1968 the Division of University Extension of the University of Delaware conducted for the Association of Delaware Hospitals a survey of educational training requirements for the supervisory and administrative personnel of the association's member institutions. The association's director of education then asked the extension division to help plan a packaged program for supervisory training; the association made this program available to individual hospitals, to order annually as a whole or in part.

Again, the first director of education of the Arizona Hospital Association offered his services as a consultant to hospital-based trainers and began a yearly audit of hospitals' training programs.

One of the first activities of the director of education of the Arkansas Hospital Association, with the cooperation of the state department of education, was to organize a program for "training the trainers" through a series of workshops that made up a 36-hour course held in six of the seven hospital districts of the state. Following these sessions, the education director provided supportive services to the trainers, recruiting faculty, publishing a newsletter, and conducting statewide and district institutes for such groups as hospital business managers, engineers, housekeepers, personnel directors, and medical record librarians.

In Wisconsin, the state association director of education, in cooperation with the extension division of the University of Wisconsin, developed and moderated nearly 60 hours of telephone and radio network programs, in both lecture and problem-solving formats, in addition to developing other audiovisual programs. The Wisconsin association also helped state vocational school districts to plan and operate circuit-riding and inhouse programs of continuing education for supervisory personnel.

When the Iowa Hospital Association began a coordinated program of continuing education, it was assigned to the association's director of hospital nursing, because in most Iowa hospitals nurses are responsible for training. In 1966, 22 Iowa hospitals had inservice educational programs; by 1970, all 145 hospitals had some type of staff development program. The association sponsored a series of district workshops to reach 6000 nurses, who received management training and instruction in leadership techniques.

The Ohio Hospital Association explored ways of defining and expanding the relationships between the educational programs of a state and a metropolitan hospital association—in this case, the Greater Cleveland Hospital Council. The educational activities of the Cleveland council previously were limited mainly to health careers recruitment. With funding from the state association, the council also entered into preemployment programs, course development, and continuing education. Negotiations with the Television Training Institute gave hospitals as a group a voice in planning telecasts that could be used for employee training within each hospital. A cooperative effort with the Cleveland Board of Education made basic instruction in the "3 R's" available to hospital employees inside the hospitals. The Ohio Hospital Association reported that its educational effectiveness was greatly increased as a result of the expanded activities in Cleveland.

Functions of the Association Director of Education

Over the last decade, regional, state, and local hospital associations have been defining their educational roles and expanding services. The most successful programs have been those in which the director of education acted as a facilitator and coordinator of services in the interest of better education and training in individual member hospitals.

Today, a realistic job description for a state association director of education should include these functions:

1. To determine the continuing education needs of personnel in member hospitals

2. To plan and coordinate programs to meet these needs

3. To identify planning and teaching resources, and to provide informational services to member hospitals

4. To cooperate with professional health care associations and with educational institutions

5. To cooperate with state and federal government agencies interested in manpower development and health care education

6. To expedite the use of public and foundation funds available for hospital education and training programs

Whether the director of education also works on recruitment programs, preservice training, and other types of personnel development depends on the size of the association staff and its financial resources. Some directors of education in the smaller associations have become involved in general association activities, such as legislative matters. These pressures are not necessarily detrimental; many seemingly extraneous activities can and do provide insight into the actual and potential contributions of educational programs.

RECOMMENDATIONS FOR DIRECTORS OF EDUCATION

Hospital associations' master plans for continuing education should reflect their long-range goals. If directors of education will begin now to plan their overall educational programs on a one-year to three-year basis, they can build continuity into their efforts. They can appraise programs, improving and recycling them according to the needs of the membership. They can conduct experimental programs and manpower studies, sharing their findings through various means of communication.

The directors of education must regularly and systematically assess the need for educational programs within and among hospitals. Decisions on what programming will be done, for whom and how it will be done, when it will be done, and who will do it, must be thought out in the context of identified needs and priorities. Surveys, interviews, and relevant publications are all useful tools. Through advisory committees, the directors of education may develop accurate estimates of the extent to which member hospitals will support a program, financially and through active participation.

Regular personal visits to hospitals are indispensable for identifying training needs and determining the kinds of programming that can best be done through the hospital association. The best way to gain the cooperation of the hospital staff is to meet them face to face in the hospital setting. Another advantage of visits to hospitals is that they provide the opportunity to identify strong educational programs and talented instructional staff who can be valuable resources for other hospitals to consult. The directors of education must seek ways to help hospitals develop and improve their orientation programs, their on-the-job training, their inservice programs, and their supervisory education. Most hospital training personnel attempt these kinds of training, and in these areas association support can be most productive. Education directors should study a sample of programs in individual hospitals and discuss them with hospital personnel in terms of their objectives, organization, and results. It will be helpful if they can suggest sound programs currently being offered elsewhere that might serve as examples for adaptation by individual hospitals.

Finally, directors of education must devise ways to measure and appraise the impact of their educational efforts. Are educational programs being developed by and for local hospitals as a result of association efforts? Is job performance being improved through on-the-job training? Are new employees receiving better orientation? Are supervisors learning the skills of administration and personnel management? The true evaluation of association efforts will be found in feedback from local hospitals.

6

Trustees: A Neglected Group

Members of hospital governing boards, no less than any other group in the hospital, have specialized continuing education needs. The Hospital Continuing Education Project staff solicited the views of 30 persons interested in hospital trustees' educational needs—hospital administrators, governing board members, and representatives of hospital associations—as an effort merely to begin a useful investigation. Our interviews confirmed the recent observation of Raymond Sloan, one of America's most knowledgeable hospital trustees, that "in terms of education, there probably is no more neglected group in a hospital than its trustees."

Trustees of today's voluntary hospital are expected to subordinate their particular interests, or the narrowly conceived interests of their single institution, to the best interests of the entire community. They must be prepared to harmonize the demands of public opinion, government, consumers, and employees with the objectives of the hospital. Changes affecting the autonomy of the hospital—unionization, the creation of health maintenance organizations, shared service programs, mergers, rate review programs—will be anticipated by board members who are aware of and who understand national health care problems and issues; the same changes, however inevitable, may appear threatening to board members accustomed to concerning themselves only with the hospital's internal operations. It is not enough to turn to the trustees in a moment of crisis to try to gain their understanding of problems facing the hospital; as long as they serve on the board, they need background education and current information on health care affairs. They also need specific factual information on the daily affairs of the hospital. For the hospital trying to educate its trustees in this way, the truth is that there are very few resources in terms of model programs, materials, or support from educational institutions or hospital associations.

EDUCATIONAL NEEDS

Legally and morally, the board of trustees is responsible for the policies and operation of the hospital, and the same factors that are steadily enlarging the scope of this responsibility also require trustees to be more knowledgeable than in the past about the field of health care. To cite the most familiar of these factors:

1. The increasing importance of the hospital as a locus for medical practice

2. The emergence of the hospital as the coordinator of community health services

3. The trend toward providing preventive as well as curative care

4. The shift in the administrator's primary function from supervising business operations to planning and developing future programs

5. The growing participation of federal and state governments in the field of health care

A broader view of its responsibilities is being forced upon the governing board through federal and state legislation, through court decisions in negligence and malpractice suits, and through activities of planning agencies. Recent court decisions have made it unmistakably clear that trustees must accept responsibility for the quality of medical care provided in the hospital; therefore, the board must understand the legal implications of its responsibility for the actions of the hospital medical staff and of personnel. The board needs to review with legal counsel statutes and court decisions applicable to granting medical staff privileges. The board must periodically reexamine the roles and duties of nurses and ancillary personnel in the light of personnel shortages, medical and technological advances, new services, and changing licensure requirements.

The board must understand and insist that the hospital implement the standards of the Joint Commission on Accreditation of Hospitals and of state licensing bodies, and should consider them as the minimum standards for medical care. The board needs to study current and proposed federal and state health care legislation, and may want to investigate appropriate means of influencing the passage of legislation.

Board members must be acquainted in some organized way with the economic, social, ethical, and legal issues that underlie hospital-physician relations nationally and in their own communities. Medicare requirements compel the board to concern itself with the workings of utilization review committees. Hospital physician-specialist relationships are central to an understanding of health care financing, and the positions of the various medical groups involved in such situations should be clear to the board. A trustee education program could profitably explore what a board can do to reduce anxiety and potential conflict between the medical staff and the board without relinquishing board responsibility.

An educational program should help trustees understand the relationship of their hospital to other health care agencies and institutions in their service area. Hospital trustees frequently are not sufficiently involved in the activities of metropolitan and regional planning agencies. Trustees from different hospitals in a community should meet together, at least informally but regularly, for mutual enlightenment, discussion of common problems, and a display of solidarity in support of a communitywide approach to health care. They may then become more interested in cooperative ventures among hospitals to provide educational and other shared services.

In brief, trustees need to be well-informed about:

1. Legal responsibilities of the board

2. Management policies of the hospital

3. Relationships between the hospital and physicians

4. Social and economic factors underlying changes in health care delivery and financing

5. Community planning for the allocation of health care resources

6. Current and proposed legislation affecting the delivery and financing of health care

In addition to this general knowledge, trustees need specific information about their own hospital in order to make policy decisions—the kind of information that will help them to pose questions regarding the allocation of resources (for new services, for example) or alternative courses of action. A basic requirement is accurate financial data, interpreted by the administrator. Trustees also need sufficient information on the utilization and costs of the various hospital services, and on the expressed needs of patients and the community, to judge whether the hospital's services are accessible to those who need them, and at the lowest possible cost. At the same time, the board must hold the medical staff responsible for demonstrating that it is maintaining and improving the quality of medical care.

ORIENTATION FOR NEW TRUSTEES

Given these real needs of the board members for preparation and continuing information, what are the responsibilities of the hospital? Many administrators recognize the need of new trustees for an intensive orientation into the unique organization of the hospital, because the management of patient care is unlike the management of any other business with which trustees may be familiar. They also need to become acquainted with many facets of modern medical care and its vocabulary. Orientation programs give new board members a comprehensive look at what the hospital is doing and help them relate their assignments to the complete range of board activities.

A hospital that is planning to start a formal trustee orientation program may apply for information or assistance to another hospital with a successful program, to local and state hospital associations, and to the American Hospital Association and the American College of Hospital Administrators. In the interest of strengthening board-administrator relations, the administrator should coordinate the program himself.

Usually orientation programs cover a planned agenda in a series of meetings. Some procedures that have proved successful are these:

1. Invite prospective trustees to sit in on a board meeting so they can gain some first-hand understanding of what the board does.

2. Provide each new trustee with an orientation manual that contains useful materials selected by the board president and the administrator. Include, for example, a history of the hospital, a copy of the hospital's charter and bylaws, an organizational chart, a description of the various departments and their functions, the hospital's most recent annual report, a description of the board committees and their functions, copies of board and board committee minutes for the last year, a copy of such pertinent medical staff documents as its bylaws, a review of the hospital's educational and research activities, and reprints of published articles useful to the trustee.

3. Bring into the orientation program board members, executive staff members, medical staff members, and community leaders who can contribute to trustee education; for example:

   • Hospital department heads, the hospital comptroller, hospital legal counsel, and the chairman of the hospital auxiliary

   • Experienced board members who can discuss informally such matters as the purposes and objectives of the hospital, the hospital's role in community affairs, long-range plans, and so forth

   • Community leaders, including trustees of other hospitals, executives of planning agencies, and metropolitan and regional hospital association executives

4. Use a variety of educational media, including films and tape cassettes, and provide subscriptions to the American Hospital Association's *Trustee, Journal for Hospital Governing Boards.*

5. Arrange tours of the hospital and of other hospitals in the vicinity.

6. Appoint new trustees to board committees toward the end of the orientation period.

RECOMMENDATIONS FOR CONTINUING EDUCATION

Providing for the continuing education of the board of trustees is more difficult than arranging an orientation program. As a matter of fact, the use of the phrase "continuing education" is offensive to some trustees. It is gratuitous, they explain, to speak of educating the board; the trustee educates himself, if given opportunities.

Board meetings, supplemented by written materials, have traditionally been the means by which the administrator keeps his board informed. Any program must conserve time for the board members, be well organized, current, and unmistakably necessary and worthwhile. Whatever written materials are used should be as brief as practicable, presented in an attractive format, and sent to board members in advance of the meetings. Accurate summaries may accompany or substitute for entire documents, because materials sent to a board member compete with his other interests for his attention.

One experienced hospital trustee, Nathan Stark, believes that the traditional role of the hospital board, in which the board merely receives monthly or quarterly reports on past performance, frustrates both the interest and the potential contribution of the trustees, and that changing the organization to give them active roles would develop trustee specialists able to deal effectively with important issues. As an example, he suggests forming temporary task forces of trustees and qualified professionals, with assistance by the administration, to work on particular problems—such as those that require adaptation to changing environment, collaboration among many groups or agencies, or intense commitment to the hospital's goals. He believes that the trustee's skills in problem solving could be put to work in this kind of organization to deal with such matters as outreach programs, neighborhood clinics, home health care, ambulatory care, medical education, and relationships with other health care institutions and agencies.

Workshops, seminars, institutes, and convention programs planned for trustees have often been poorly attended. Some trustees, explaining that they have little time for attending meetings, suggest that an administrator attend meetings and summarize the proceedings for the board, while others complain that institute faculties are usually dominated by administrators. Many support the idea of local one-day workshops and local informational sessions with members of the staffs of state hospital associations, who might travel through the state to meet with hospital trustees. State hospital associations that have planned educational workshops have had uneven results. It may be significant that one association attributes its success to the continued involvement of governing board members in designing programs planned for them, while another association, distressed by the small attendance at its trustee workshops, acknowledges that one reason might have been the fact that administrators and association personnel planned the programs for trustees "who wouldn't know what issues it was important for them to understand."

Perhaps trustees would attend meetings of only one or two days, for which expenses would be paid by the hospital, where faculty with recognized expertise—whether university professors, other trustees, businessmen, executives of hospital associations or government agencies—could offer useful and otherwise unavailable educational experiences. Workshops for trustees might be conducted at regular intervals by university graduate programs in health care administration and by university centers for continuing education. The academic setting appeals to many trustees, who are familiar with the idea of continuing education for business executives in a university setting.

Many local and individual efforts for trustee orientation and continuing education have been successful. But the burden of locating resources, planning programs, and devising techniques for keeping the board informed has rested almost entirely on the individual administrator and his staff, who have had little or no opportunity for systematic experimentation or for profiting from one another's experience. There has been little imaginative use of modern educational technology or of educational resources outside the hospital to create comprehensive educational programs for trustees.

One example of the creative use of educational technology for the benefit of hospital governing board members is the series of audio tape cassettes, *Tapes for Trustees,* offered by the Hospital Research and Educational Trust. These tapes, which the Trust developed in cooperation with Teach'em, Inc., of Chicago, carry informal conversations with health care leaders on subjects requested by board members: health care trends, legal responsibilities of the board, trustee-medical staff relationships, trustee-administrator relationships, and so forth. The cassettes may be played by the trustee at any convenient time or place, and are being used for both individual and group education. Another example of taped programs for trustees is a series of 11 video tapes that was recently produced by the South Carolina Hospital Association with funding by the South Carolina Regional Medical Program. The 15-minute cassettes feature speakers who give brief talks on state and national health care issues affecting local hospitals and then answer questions from a panel of hospital administrators and trustees.

Although national resources must be brought to bear in the development of such programs, it is fatuous to believe that national organizations can do more than provide encouragement, identify issues, offer faculty, and develop educational materials to be used on a regional, local, or institutional basis. To attract trustees to educational meetings beyond convenient geographical limits is unworkable, except in the most extraordinary circumstances.

Therefore, the question is how to develop programs that bring trustees together locally or that use the still relatively new educational tools, such as the audio cassette, to bring information to the trustee in the most convenient manner, making it easier for him to reserve time from his busy schedule for keeping up with health care developments. The experience of universities in the East, Midwest, and West indicates that trustees are receptive to personal invitations from presidents of universities and colleges to participate in one-day programs developed in concert with hospital organizations. One university, working with hospital associations in a number of states, has begun to develop a regional program. Another state hospital organization has conceived a plan for dividing the state into districts for trustee education, with hospital administrators acting as staff and resources for trustees in each district.

It will take this type of experimentation over the next few years, with appropriate evaluation, to arrive at models for trustee education. What is needed is a continuing education program using nationally developed guides and other teaching materials, but applied locally in a manner that is sensitive to both local issues and local patterns for reaching the trustee.

7

Administrators, Department Managers, and Supervisors

MEETING ADMINISTRATORS' NEEDS

At first glance, it would seem that the needs of hospital administrators for learning experiences distributed throughout their working lives not only are recognized by universities and professional associations, but are well supplied through a host of publications, institutes, and convention programs. There is little doubt that most administrators try to keep abreast of current problems and to improve their management capabilities by pursuing their own continuing education through reading, discussions with colleagues, and taking advantage of meetings and institutes. For example, nearly 70 percent of the more than 400 midwestern hospital administrators responding to a survey conducted in 1965 by the St. Louis University Center for Hospital Continuing Education, and more than 85 percent of the 268 administrators responding to a survey conducted by the New England Center for Continuing Education in 1969, reported having attended one or more educational programs in the two years preceding the surveys. What has been less clear is whether the various sources of continuing education for hospital administrators are actually meeting their needs.

Survey of Administrators' Needs

To answer this question, it seems essential to know how hospital administrators perceive their own continuing education needs and what they recommend for suitable continuing education programs. At the start of 1973, two groups of hospital executives selected from the membership roster of the American College of Hospital Administrators were surveyed. Selection was random except for age: one group consisted of 200 persons 47 to 48 years old, and the other of 200 persons 31 to 32 years old. All were working in hospitals at that time, the younger group generally in junior executive capacities (assistant administrators), and the older group generally in senior executive capacities (chief executive officers). The response rate for the junior group was 59 percent, and for the senior executives, 49 percent.

Content Areas of Interest

The questionnaire (Appendix B) contained two sections. The first listed 14 content areas or topics, and the administrators were asked to indicate those they had studied in the last two years, and to rank in order of priority those which they personally would like for their further continuing education. The responses (Table 23, next page) indicated that the number who had availed themselves of continuing education was slightly greater for the senior group of administrators than for the junior group. However, the content area ranked highest by both the older and the younger group, in terms of both past study and continuing interest, was financial management.[1]

When the content areas studied in the past two years are ranked in order of frequency checked, the ranking tends to be similar for both groups in all instances except three. The ranking of governing board relations and of medical staff relations was higher for the senior executives, while the ranking of organizational theory was higher for the junior executives.

In regard to interest in future study, both groups gave high priority to financial management, medical staff relations, and institutional planning. On the other hand, both groups gave low priority to further study of fund raising, psychology, and sociology. Apart from these areas of agreement, there were the following differences: legal problems were ranked second by junior executives, but fifth by senior executives, and the juniors were more interested than the seniors in studying economics and design and construction. Governing board relations ranked third among areas of continuing interest for the senior executives, but only eighth as an interest of the junior group, and the seniors also showed more interest in studying personnel administration.

Sources Used for Continuing Education

The second section of the survey was designed to find out what sources these administrators would prefer to use to meet their stated educational needs, as well as to find out the sources they actually had used in the previous two years (Table 24, next page). The sources listed were classroom programs, such as institutes and evening classes; individual reading; self-instructional materials, including audio cassettes, correspondence courses, and television; and conventions, sabbatical leaves for study, and study tours. In interpreting the responses, it must be remembered that certain sources may have been too remote or too expensive to use. The responses

---

1. The earlier regional surveys also stressed this need. The 1965 study of the continuing education needs of administrative personnel in midwestern hospitals by the St. Louis University Center for Hospital Continuing Education found that finances ranked second among the management problems reported. In the 1969 survey by the New England Hospital Assembly, study of financial management ranked second among the educational needs expressed by hospital administrators in that region.

Table 23. Specified Content Areas Studied by Senior and Junior Executive Officers During 1971-72, and/or of Interest to Them for Future Study

Content Area	Studied in Past Two Years				Rank Order of Interest for Future Study	
	SEO* (N=98)		JEO** (N=118)		SEO	JEO
	Percent	Rank Order	Percent	Rank Order		
Financial management	60	1	48	1	1	1
Medical staff relations	59	2	39	4	2	3
Legal problems	51	3	48	2	5	2
Governing board relations	47	4	16	11	3	8
Personnel administration	39	5	33	6	6	10
Design and construction	34	6	37	5	11	7
Institutional planning	34	7	30	8	4	4
Management engineering	33	8	32	7	8	9
Economics	32	9	27	9	9	6
Organizational theory	30	10	47	3	7	5
Education and training	26	11	27	10	10	11
Fund raising	10	12	11	12	13	12
Psychology	6	13	9	13	12	13
Sociology	2	14	8	14	14	14

*Random sample of 98 senior executive officers (47 to 48 years old).
**Random sample of 118 junior executive officers (31 to 32 years old).

Table 24. Specified Sources for Continuing Education Used During 1971-72 by Senior and Junior Executive Officers, and/or Preferred by Them

Source	Sources Used in Past Two Years				Sources Preferred			
	SEO*		JEO**		SEO		JEO	
	Percent	Rank Order	Percent	Rank Order	Percent	Rank Order	Percent	Rank Order
Journals	97	1	96	1	60	3	56	2
Newsletters	94	2	94	2	56	4	47	4
Institutes	91	3	90	3	82	1	82	1
Conventions	91	4	90	4	51	5	40	6
Books	83	5	82	5	41	6	56	3
Audio cassettes	69	6	47	6	62	2	43	5
Evening courses	10	7	18	7	26	9	29	7
Television	10	8	15	8	19	10	20	10
Correspondence	5	9	8	10	15	11	17	11
Study tours	—	—	9	9	31	7	23	8
Leaves	—	—	—	—	30	8	24	9

*Random sample of 98 senior executive officers (47 to 48 years old).
**Random sample of 118 junior executive officers (31 to 32 years old).

indicate which of the listed sources were used, but do not indicate which were available as realistic choices.

It is interesting that the outstanding preference of both groups was for institutes. There are no major differences apparent between the two groups of respondents in the rankings of sources actually used. Over 90 percent of both groups indicated that in the previous two years they had used journals, newsletters, institutes, and conventions for continuing education, in that order. Over 80 percent of both groups had read books for professional education. Although both groups ranked audio cassettes sixth among sources used, about 70 percent of the senior executive group had used cassettes, in contrast to about 50 percent of the junior executive group. Less than 10 percent of both groups had used correspondence courses.

There is some indication that certain differences in the preferences of these administrators for continuing education sources may be related to the effects of age or of age and position, although the questionnaire was not designed to measure these effects precisely.

In answer to the question of what sources would be preferred for continuing education, the respondents did not need to consider the availability of the sources, and they could take into account their past satisfaction or dissatisfaction with the sources on the list. Institutes and audio cassettes ranked higher in terms of preference than in terms of past use. However, individual reading sources—journals, newsletters, and books—all ranked lower in the list of preferences than in the list of sources used. Although publications are a ready source of education, the respondents may find that those available do not fulfill their personal needs, or they may prefer more structured study in certain content areas.

Evening courses, television, and correspondence courses ranked low in terms of both use and preference. Although the use of these sources is affected by availability, the responses in terms of preference indicated that greater availability still might not have promoted greater use. However, it should be noted that the structured programs described earlier, which combine home study with university classes and personal guidance from faculty and preceptors, have been well received where they have been offered.

The overall implications of the responses may be summed up as follows: the traditionally used and readily available sources of continuing education are not really fulfilling the perceived needs of these administrators. Certainly, the preferences expressed for institutes and for audio cassettes (especially on the part of the older executives, who reported more previous experience in using cassettes) suggest that administrators prefer structured and convenient study opportunities. Many of the write-in comments on the questionnaires stressed the advantages of other learning situations, such as institutes, that make possible personal exchanges of ideas. It is probable, however, that satisfaction with continuing education opportunities is due as much to a satisfactory choice of subject matter as to the sources used. Opportunities for continuing education that are new in regard to both sources and subject matter may be called for.

New Directions for Continuing Education

The responses of practicing administrators to the questionnaire indicate that there is a need to reevaluate (1) the sources of continuing education currently available and (2) the material conveyed through these sources. There are indications that the present range of opportunities for continuing education for administrators is not meeting their needs for convenience, for organized study of the topics most urgently demanding their attention, or for personal give-and-take with their colleagues and with other experts.

The content areas in which the survey respondents would most like continuing education are financial management, medical staff relations, institutional planning, governing board relations (third choice of the senior executives), and legal problems (second choice of the junior executives). These choices obviously reflect both the perennial concerns of the administrator and the current economic and social pressures on the hospital. Health care institutions and organizations are changing and will continue to change in response to these pressures, and they will need administrators with a new orientation and new skills.

The greater attention now being given to the management of health services finds our health care system short—both quantitatively and qualitatively—of adequately prepared managers. Continuing education programs can contribute both to developing greater numbers of health care managers and to improving their preparation. Administrators need a broader program of studies, including certain topics that may not have been suggested to the survey respondents by the content areas specified in the questionnaire. Both prospective and practicing administrators also need more alternatives to full-time programs for obtaining graduate school education, which is becoming the union card for hospital administration. As the discussion of the format combining residential study and home study pointed out, the majority of hospital administrators, and probably most administrators of small hospitals, have not had formal graduate education in hospital administration.[2] More continuing education opportunities are needed for these administrators.

Community-oriented Education

Today, the public—as community, constituents, or consumers—is demanding to participate in the direction of hospitals and all other major institutions of our society, and the forces represented by these demands are here to stay. Consumer groups developing new mechanisms for the delivery of health care sometimes disregard the hospital and all of its capability and experience, because of what they interpret as its lack of concern or understanding. Even as this is happening, health care administrators who are trying to consolidate control of the rapidly growing and complex hospital organization and to improve the businesslike efficiency of its management may underestimate the potential benefits of community participation in formulating institutional policies. Administrators need to have understanding of the social forces affecting the hospital, familiarity with the motivation and the working methods of community groups making demands upon the hospital, and skill in dealing with relationships between such groups and the hospital.

Recognizing the significance of social changes, universities have been acting to broaden the preparation of administrators by offering programs in health services administration, rather than restricting their programs to hospital administration. They

---

2. The 1965 survey of hospital administrators by the St. Louis University Center for Hospital Continuing Education showed that over 90 percent of the respondents in hospitals with fewer than 100 beds did not have graduate-level education in hospital administration, while half of the respondents in hospitals with more than 100 beds were graduates of master's degree programs. Large hospitals employed more administrators with previous administrative experience and training, while small hospitals employed more administrators promoted from within. The New England Hospital Assembly survey of administrators' educational needs in 1969 also concluded that the "less highly educated tend to manage the smaller facilities."

are expanding the size of their student bodies to meet the need for more managers, and they are gearing their curriculums to the development of administrators who will have breadth of view and the capacity for foresight and initiative, as well as the necessary practical skills.

The need to develop community-oriented administrative skills and understanding is equally important for continuing education programs. It has been suggested that there may be no classroom substitute for direct experience in working with consumer groups, and that both preparatory and continuing education should offer this kind of experience. Administrators who were prepared in a more narrowly conceived curriculum need continuing education that will help them deal with community relations problems confronting the health care system at the present time.

Minorities and Career Mobility

If the health care field is to assemble the managerial manpower that it needs today, it must develop all of its human resources. In a recent discussion of the need for a more aggressive national program to help minorities gain their rightful places in managerial and administrative posts in the health care field, it was pointed out that as long as minorities do not have this opportunity, the nation's health care system—as well as the aspiring worker—loses. The system loses because, although it serves all sorts of minority populations, it will not have in key administrative positions the people most sensitive to the needs and demands of those populations. Hospitals without minority representation on their administrative staffs may deny themselves a point of view that they need to be responsive to their communities.

What kinds of continuing education would create more access routes for health care personnel to rise to managerial positions? Staff development programs in large hospitals, or programs sponsored on a shared basis by a number of hospitals? University courses offered in late afternoons, evenings, or on weekends? Members of minority groups, including women, now constitute a large proportion of hospital personnel. Among the constraints to attracting them into health care administration have been the length and rigidity of the curriculums. If opportunities were available, health care personnel could attend classes part time while remaining on the job. Universities with health services administration programs are increasingly recognizing that they have a responsibility to become more flexible, and to make their services available to those unable to take advantage of full-time programs. Enlightened employers might find it a good long-term investment to defray part of such educational expenses.

In looking at the matter of career mobility as it relates to minority aspirations, it is important to remember that from the minority point of view the staff development route may be considered a second-class approach, in contrast to the first-class university route that has been the path of others toward administrative appointments. It has also been pointed out that although promotion from within is to be encouraged, it may lead to an assistant-administrator position in one hospital but may not be translatable into a top administrative post in another hospital. Innovative programs are needed, not only to increase minority representation among graduate students in health services administration but also to provide new approaches to the continuing education of those who have proven themselves in departmental assignments, to enable them to qualify for higher and more general administrative responsibilities.

SUPERVISORY DEVELOPMENT

Supervisors and department heads make up the majority of the hospital management force. Their urgent need for better training in the theory and techniques of management appeared as a common theme in the surveys of educational needs conducted as part of the Hospital Continuing Education Project by the Association of Delaware Hospitals, the University of Alabama, the University of Minnesota and the New England Hospital Assembly.[3] Also, in the survey of hospital-based trainers (Chapter 2), supervisory training shared top ranking with continuing education on the list of training needs expected to increase; 79 percent of the respondents predicted that the need for supervisory development would increase in their hospitals in the following two years.

The same concern has been widely expressed and documented elsewhere. A study of hospital personnel problems, conducted at St. Vincent's Hospital in New York City and funded by the U.S. Department of Health, Education, and Welfare, recommended clearing up misunderstandings between supervisors and department heads in regard to the supervisors' responsibility and authority. A study of personnel turnover conducted by the United Hospital Fund of New York commented: "A basic weakness that appears in every depth analysis of the causes of turnover in hospitals is the weakness of ineffective supervision and management, which manifests itself in a lack of employee training and motivation. . . . The main causes of avoidable turnover are therefore perpetuated because of inadequate staff—both in numbers and in competence to perform and grow in self-direction."

Shortcomings of Supervisory Training Efforts

Many administrators are not cognizant of their own important role in the development of subordinates, and devote little, if any, time to it. Often, attendance of a supervisor or department head at a training institute is offered as a reward in itself, and little is expected in the way of feedback or sharing of the learning experience.

Most supervisory training is offered through short institutes, workshops, and conferences. Transfer of learning from these experiences to the job is difficult, because their stimulus is short-lived and no follow-up is possible. In the case of university or college-based supervisory training courses, the learning period is extended, but it is still nearly impossible for the instructor to do any follow-up work with the student, and some instructors are only casually familiar with hospital organization and prob-

---

3. The recommendations of the 1968 survey of educational and training requirements for supervisory/administrative personnel of the member institutions of the Association of Delaware Hospitals corroborate the criteria for optimum supervisory training suggested here. The report stated that supervisory personnel needed most a course in personnel management, and secondly, a course in planning—fiscal, personnel, and work planning. The report recommended that brief versions of the courses offered to supervisors be presented to the administrators as a group, and that classes combine supervisory personnel from grouped hospitals. In regard to methods and materials, the report recommended using group participation methods rather than formal lectures, and using educational television when a qualified leader could be found to lead discussion after each telecast.

lems. In either short institutes or longer on-campus programs, only a few supervisors from any one institution may participate at one time. Although they may indeed achieve new skills, they often find it difficult to use these skills because of resistance from their peers and superiors who do not share their new insights.

Supervisory training materials directly related to the hospital setting are scarce; more often than not, case studies are drawn from industry. With few exceptions, the hospital and health care field has failed to develop and circulate supervisory training materials of high quality.

Furthermore, much of the course content in existing training programs is concept-oriented, and the student is expected to figure out how to apply the concepts to his job. The present trend in the teaching of management is to consider management as a group of processes rather than as a system of concepts.

Future supervisory training should take account of these recognized shortcomings of many past efforts—administrative neglect, inadequate materials, and the difficulty of transferring learning from the classroom to the job.

Models for Supervisory Training

There is need for a variety of models for supervisory training that can be adapted to local circumstances and used by hospital directors of education and training, or by instructors in community colleges, vocational schools, and universities that co-operate with hospitals and hospital associations. The supervisory training programs developed by the University of Minnesota and by the Association of Delaware Hospitals, which have been noted in Chapters 4 and 5, exemplify the kind of experimentation needed.[4] To suggest another experimental model, the residential–home-study format described in Chapter 4 as a vehicle of continuing education for administrators may prove useful for offering hospital department managers an educational experience that cannot be duplicated by short-term courses.

The first goal of supervisory training should be to satisfy the basic needs of the supervisor to understand the specific responsibilities for which he is accountable, and to become competent in carrying out these responsibilities. The supervisor will be more receptive to continuing education when he is confident not only of his competence in the performance of his tasks, but also of his ability to train and to support those he supervises in their tasks, and to create a climate conducive to experimentation and improvement.

---

4. Another example is a television training series for supervisory personnel in hospitals, co-sponsored by the United Hospital Fund of New York and the Greater New York Hospital Association, that was broadcast in New York City from January through May of 1966. In order to make this supervisory training available to a wider audience, the Hospital Continuing Education Project granted funds for the transfer of the video tape to motion picture film and for the evaluation of the series by the Office of Research and Evaluation Services of the School of Education, College of the City of New York. A procedure similar to that recommended in Delaware was followed in New York; after each of the five televised presentations, an appointed leader in each hospital conducted a discussion with the viewing supervisors and distributed supplementary materials, which the viewers found very useful. However, it appeared that a half-hour television program once a month was more successful in improving insight than in teaching techniques of management.

In designing model supervisory training programs the following considerations should be taken into account:

1. *Supervisory development programs should be planned as long-term programs with logical continuity.* Programs should be planned in multiple modular units, and should be designed so that existing delivery systems can be utilized for implementation. The basic module should be related to the basic needs described above, with subsequent modules so related that any single module may be selected to meet immediate specific needs of the supervisors.

2. *Working groups should be recognized as the target groups for supervisory training.* Program design should encourage the training of organic groups; an effort should be made to train together at least the supervisors in a single department or in related departments. The whole group of supervisors could then move together in one developing frame of reference.

   Multiple levels of management must also be involved. The supervisors' superiors at the next two higher levels should be brought into the picture in some way, so that all clearly understand their roles, responsibilities, and objectives.

   Program design should help the administrator to perform his appropriate role in supervisory development. Without his participation, it is unlikely that any lasting change will occur in the management behavior of the hospital.

3. *The content of model training programs should be job-oriented.* Taking the point of view that supervisory development means training in the processes of managing, the first consideration should be the work that the supervisor must perform each day, and the relationship of his performance to the attitudes and performance of his subordinates. In order to understand the tasks for which he is accountable, the supervisor needs:

   - To know the nature and quality of results expected of him;

   - To know specifically what authority has been delegated to him;

   - To know and understand hospital policies that have a bearing on his role;

   - To be aware of the impact of his work group's output on other departments and on patients; and

   - To understand the effect of his performance on the effectiveness of his work group.

   Content should emphasize goal setting, the identification by the supervisor of specific tasks in which his performance may be improved, and processes that will lead to improvement.

4. *Educational materials should be developed and tested.* They should be relevant to the hospital and use current educational methods and teaching aids.

Opportunities for Advancement

The present work force in the health care field offers an excellent source of undeveloped administrative talent. It is important to remember that tomorrow's administrators may come from today's department heads as well as from graduate programs, and that staff development programs may be the training ground for tomorrow's department managers. People currently holding jobs in the health care field need continuing education opportunities to prepare for advancement to department management or to general administration. Although their educational opportunities may have been limited, these people have already established their major interest in health care, and an evaluation of their job performance would indicate those with real potential for advancement. Attempts in this direction might offer them a way out of dead-end jobs, and for hospitals, might open a needed source of administrative manpower.

8

Educational Technology[1]

The health care field must take better advantage of new technology in training and education. Even though the uses of new audiovisual aids and teaching techniques have been demonstrated, their potential for health care education has yet to be realized. Here, the federal government has an opportunity to join voluntary organizations and the burgeoning educational industry in a massive effort directed especially toward training in health care skills. Innovations are essential if the health care field is to solve the problem of bringing education and training programs of high quality to its large and decentralized work force.

Educational and health care institutions should work jointly with private industry, drawing on its experience in research and development and in distributing its products. But quantity production of new equipment and teaching materials is not the whole answer to the needs of health care educators. In fact, competitive development of new audiovisual products has led to a proliferation of hardware and software with little standardization, so that one manufacturer's film cartridge will not fit into another manufacturer's projector. Industry can make a major contribution by taking an active part in developing new methods of learning and teaching, and above all, in working out new systems that combine different types of educational equipment and methods.

There will never be enough instructors to meet the continuing education needs of health services personnel if instructors continue to rely mainly on traditional training

---

1. This chapter was prepared in collaboration with Jerome P. Lysaught, Ed.D., Professor of Education and Professor of Medical Education at the University of Rochester, Rochester, N.Y.

methods. Even though the effectiveness of some innovations may still be uncertain, new methods must be tried. It should be possible to extend the reach of the hospital personnel who are available as instructors by making use of audiovisual aids and self-instructional methods, which disregard traditional distinctions between teachers and learners.

SELF-INSTRUCTIONAL LEARNING

The story of programmed or self-instructional learning as it is used today began in the fall of 1958, when B. F. Skinner, the behavioral psychologist, offered his Harvard students the first "learning program." Based on his previous experiments with lower organisms, it was Skinner's belief that the essential element in learning is feedback, or the immediate discovery by the learner that his response is correct or incorrect.

A programmed course of instruction may be reproduced on paper or presented to the learner by a teaching machine; in either case, it must clearly state objectives and divide the instructional content required to reach these objectives into a series of steps that the learner takes one by one. Each step (frame) consists of a question (stimulus); the learner's answer (response); and the feedback (confirmation). As the learner proceeds, responding to every question and repeating the material until he masters it, his incorrect responses are extinguished when he discovers his errors, and his correct responses are reinforced as he finds that they are right. Material developed in this way, Skinner hypothesized, would permit the student to learn at his own optimum rate of speed, with minimal need for lectures or other traditional approaches to instruction. The learning program, as a "technological tutor," would facilitate self-teaching by the student.

What might otherwise have seemed to be just another professor's queer idea stirred international interest when Skinner's students did precisely as he had predicted. Without classroom lectures or outside reading, but working individually at widely varying rates of speed, all of the students passed the final examination, with their average grade recorded as one of the highest ever attained in that course. With the effectiveness of programmed learning demonstrated so clearly in a controlled experiment, it was only a matter of time before the health care professions began to explore the possibilities of adapting it to their curriculums.

In 1961, the Dartmouth Medical School Project in Self-Instruction was launched as the first formal effort to teach medical subject matter with programmed materials. This was followed in the next year by a series of projects at the University of Illinois, the University of Rochester, and the University of Southern California. Simultaneously, experimental programming was begun in nursing education and in the instruction of health technicians, technologists, and allied health workers. Interest in these experimental developments quite naturally led to a desire in the field of health care for some kind of information and data exchange. In 1963, the Office of Medical Education at the University of Rochester School of Medicine and Dentistry volunteered to provide an informational service for medical schools, and in 1966, the Hospital Continuing Education Project agreed to support a new Rochester Clearinghouse on Self-Instructional Materials for Health Care Facilities.

The response of the field to the opening of the Clearinghouse confirmed the project staff's estimate of the great latent interest in this new teaching technique. The Clearinghouse conducted five national conferences on the uses of self-instructional programs in health care education; published the proceedings of these conferences; distributed a periodic newsletter to more than 2000 subscribers; and provided a series of bibliographies, reviews, and commentaries on the applications of self-instruction to health care education. Since the termination of grant support, the University of Rochester has continued to operate the Clearinghouse as part of its activities in educational technology.[2]

The Rochester Clearinghouse has played a unique role in receiving, analyzing, and transmitting information on the developing science of instructional technology as it applies to health care education. The director, Jerome P. Lysaught, Ed.D., has formulated, from the data collected, a series of generalizations about the impact of self-instructional programs in this area. These conclusions, which are widely applicable to all kinds of health care facilities, students, and subject matter, may be stated as follows:

1. Self-instructional programs are effective.

2. Self-instructional programs are efficient.

3. Programmed instruction is accepted by the learners using it.

4. In developing self-instructional programs, the teacher may improve his skills in the educational processes of planning, teaching, and evaluation.

5. There is a wide variety of curricular uses for programmed instruction.

6. The use of programmed instruction may lead to an increase in the competence of allied health professionals and nonprofessional health care personnel.

Efficacy and Efficiency

Because self-instructional programs are constructed to attain explicitly stated goals, it might be inferred that they should successfully attain those ends. Inference, however, is not the same as evidence. In the first use of programmed instruction for medical education, at the Dartmouth Medical School, students using a self-instructional program in parasitology attained significantly higher scores on achievement tests than did matched students taught by the lecture method. In both programs, the goals of instruction and the tests were the same; the difference lay in the greater effectiveness of the programmed content. Similar conclusions were reached in research in patient education at the Cleveland Clinic, and in an extensive study involving several instructors teaching different subjects, at three institutions, carried out by the Office of Research in Medical Education at the University of Illinois.

---

2. The newsletter was suspended when the newly formed Health Sciences Communications Association announced its plan to publish an interdisciplinary journal that would treat all areas of health education and communications. Pending development of that publication, the Clearinghouse continues to supply bibliographic assistance and back issues of the newsletters and conference proceedings, but will not undertake new operations. Should the new journal not materialize, or should it not be directed, in part, to meeting the needs of health care facilities to continue exploration of self-instruction, then the Clearinghouse might resume its earlier work.

The evaluative studies of the Rochester Clearinghouse, which attempted to assess both published and unpublished but documented reports on the use of self-instructional programs in the field of medicine, found that in 66 percent of the cases reported, self-instruction was significantly superior to traditional approaches, and in an additional 30 percent of the instances, self-instruction was equal in effectiveness to conventional methods. In only 4 percent of the experiments was self-instruction found clearly less effective.[3]

A survey of programmed self-instruction in allied health education was carried out at the request of the Clearinghouse by the Office of Education at the Harvard University School of Public Health. After extensive examination of experiments in programmed learning among health care workers—laboratory technicians, technologists, and nurses—it was reported that the preponderance of evidence clearly indicated that such materials were effective over a broad range of subjects and students, and generally were more effective than any of the more traditional methods of teaching.[4]

One of the great problems in all health care education is that of efficient use of time. With so much to learn, and with the competing demands of service and operation, time is precious. For this reason, the effectiveness of programmed instruction must be considered in relation to its efficiency. Although it is easy to assume that programmed instruction must be effective, it is also seemingly natural to assume that any instructional approach that allows students to set their own pace is likely to be very inefficient. On the other hand, Skinner argued that the reinforcement provided by knowing that one's progress is successful should hasten, rather than impede, one's learning activity; and the evidence appears to bear out his argument when allowances are made for individual differences in the rate of learning.

The Dartmouth study group found that its positive results in terms of effectiveness were closely paralleled by an increased efficiency among the students using programmed instruction. In both the Clearinghouse and the Harvard surveys, there was considerable evidence that use of self-instructional programs was most often accompanied by an actual reduction in average student learning time, but with wide variations in rates of completion. Other studies have found that students using self-instructional programs took significantly less time to master given material than their counterparts who learned through classroom lectures and other conventional methods.

Acceptability to Students

Despite their effectiveness and efficiency, self-instructional materials would be of little use in health care education if they were disliked by students. Many early critics fastened on the supposed impersonality and inhumanity of self-instructional programs, in contrast to the living laboratory of the classroom, although Skinner proposed that programmed instruction might be more humane, because it was unbiased toward individual students and allowed for variable rates of learning. Studies of the use of

3. Jerome P. Lysaught, Research on self-instruction: summary and generalizations, in *Individualized Instruction in Medical Education: Proceedings of the Third Rochester Conference,* ed. Jerome P. Lysaught (Rochester, N.Y.: The Rochester Clearinghouse, 1968), p. 24.

4. L. Vanderschmidt, Programmed instruction for community medicine and public health: a selective review, in *Instructional Systems in Medical Education: Proceedings of the Fourth Rochester Conference,* ed. Jerome P. Lysaught (Rochester, N.Y.: The Rochester Clearinghouse, 1970), p. 201.

programmed instruction on the subjects of allergy and hypersensitivity, anatomy, psychiatry, microbiology, and nursing fundamentals found that students emphatically preferred the self-instructional materials to conventional lectures and readings. Among the reasons cited for this preference were the self-pacing feature of programmed self-instruction, its clarity of goals, its use of illustrations and examples, and its immediate signaling of the accuracy or inaccuracy of each response.

Although the general reaction has been favorable, there have been indications that a limited number of students definitely dislike self-instructional materials. They may simply prefer conventional teaching, or they may be discouraged by the coupling of self-instructional materials with teaching machines or other presentation devices with which they are not familiar. Negative reactions may be reduced as the use of the programmed technique becomes more common.

Many researchers have noted certain aspects of students' attitudes toward programmed materials that are as important as simple acceptance. A study of student use of a self-instructional program in hematology concluded that the learners accepted more than usual responsibility for their own learning and, on examination, performed well when required to apply cognitive learning to clinical analysis. In apparent consistency with this report, both the Clearinghouse and the Harvard surveys frequently mentioned "increased student motivation" and "heightened responsibility." It appears that students are not only willing to accept self-instructional programs, but that they become committed to learning because of their increased overt participation in the instructional process.

Improving Teaching Techniques

From the instructor's point of view, there are no unique requirements for planning self-instructional programs. However, every decision in planning programmed instruction must be made explicit and must be recorded. If any of the steps in programming are slighted, the gap becomes readily apparent. Therefore, in developing programs, instructors must make an effort to put long-accepted principles into actual practice. For example, the programming process requires that the instructor truly examine the students—individually and collectively. Although instructors know that there are wide variations in ability within any group of health care workers, they often base a lecture to a group of aides, for example, on an expectation that the result will be consistent achievement. In using programmed instruction, instructors must attempt to assess the differences among students and to provide for them. It is consistently found that, given the variations in students' learning times, the use of self-instructional programs tends to eliminate failures and to ensure that the range between the lowest and highest scores attained by students in a class is much narrower than is the case in conventional instruction.

The need to state clearly what is to be included in a self-instructional program also eliminates much haziness about objectives. Educators and trainers may fail to recognize their real differences of opinion until they are faced with developing clear objectives for a programmed course.

Developing a self-instructional program is a learning experience in itself. Instructors who have had this experience have reported that their classroom behavior has changed —more questioning, more reinforcement, and clearer specification of objectives—and that their teaching under conventional circumstances therefore has become more effective. It is significant that in one large-scale evaluation of the use of programmed instruction, the one instance in which conventional classroom teaching was as effective as the use of self-instructional materials covering the same subject was that in which the programmer turned lecturer and taught his own course.

These findings and others examined by the Clearinghouse would suggest that programmed instruction has important side effects on the development of instructional goals, on the behavior of students and faculty, and on the evaluation of results.

Versatility of Programmed Instruction

Because the first self-instructional programs in health care generally taught information, or cognitive subjects, there was suspicion that programmed instruction would have only limited application to other kinds of subject matter. By 1965, however, the majority of new self-instructional programs in health care were in the clinical areas, which involve judgment in the diagnosis, prognosis, and management of patient care.[5] Many programs designed for nonprofessional workers in the hospital have units on motor skills, including the use of equipment, the proper cleaning of areas, and the preparation of foods. These programs were designed for use with actual apparatus, so that the learner not only sees a model, but practices with the appropriate implements. A number of programs designed for patients include practice in testing urine, arranging menus, and other kinds of direct use of materials and equipment. The simulation of desired behavior is one of the many kinds of learning processes afforded by self-instructional programs. The combination of concrete and abstract learning in many self-instructional programs has demonstrated the versatility of programmed instruction.

Most self-instructional programs in subjects related to health care are relatively short sequences with circumscribed objectives. This characteristic makes it possible to use the programs in a wide variety of curriculums while maintaining instructional excellence. For example, some of the programs designed for medical technology students have been used for continuing and remedial education as well as for initial preparation, and they have also been used in teaching medical students and nurses. Just as a number of academic self-instructional programs in the behavioral and physical sciences may lend themselves to the instruction of health care practitioners, so many of the programs originally designed for medical students, nurses, or other learners may be useful for consumer education or patient self-care.

The expansion of self-instructional techniques into the area of patient care has been encouraging, as patients have responded effectively and positively to reinforced learning. Already there is broadening use of medical and nursing materials, sometimes with appropriate modifications, in the education and training of technicians, aides, and semiprofessional workers. This work has demonstrated that many so-called educational "ceilings" may be dependent on teaching techniques, rather than on innate student capacity. With the provision of variable learning times, many technicians

---

5. A bibliography of publications and programmed units (as well as a discussion of the application of programmed instruction to the hospital field) is contained in *Programmed Instruction and the Hospital; A Report on the Use of Programmed Instruction in Health Care Institutions* (Chicago: Hospital Research and Educational Trust, 1967). This publication is now out of print but is available in many libraries.

have been able to learn effectively from self-instructional programs designed for medical students. Preliminary investigation in the use of programmed instruction to develop increased competency among nonprofessional hospital employees has also been encouraging. The use of programmed self-instruction may help to expand opportunities for career mobility and advancement.

As more self-instructional materials are made available, their curricular uses will become more flexible. Instead of being tied to a lock-step approach to education and training, students will be encouraged to use materials in sequences that make the most sense in terms of their personal educational needs. Nor is programmed learning incompatible with traditional classroom instruction; it is possible to combine methods and to employ those programmed materials that are available and useful while using traditional teaching in other areas.

No one would claim that any one educational technique or method is a panacea for the problems confronting educators and trainers in the field of health care. Unlike other approaches, however, programmed materials intrinsically provide their own laboratory for development and their own methods for evaluation. When they work, it is clear that the learners have achieved. Just as important, when they fail, the situation can be examined and corrective action can be taken. To the extent that self-instructional programs can meet some immediate needs and can alleviate a number of problems, training directors can turn their attention to other unmet needs and unfulfilled objectives.

Locating and Developing Programs

There are now available well over 200 self-instructional programs in the field of health care. If one includes the number of self-instructional materials in related fields—chemistry, biology, statistics, communications, psychology, and many others—that are important in the preparatory or continuing education of health care practitioners, there are literally thousands of programs. The Rochester Clearinghouse has attempted to provide systematically updated information about these materials by listing in its own bibliography an annotated directory of other bibliographies available to health care educators and trainers. It is patently impossible for one bibliography to cover the several thousand occupational fields that are commonly found in the American health care system. By using various academic, occupational, and commercial directories, however, one may hope to scan the panorama of available materials.

Over 60 percent of the hospital-based trainers responding to the national survey discussed in Chapter 2 had used programmed instructional materials from commercial sources, but only 21 percent had developed their own programmed materials. Perhaps the latter figure should become larger. Despite the numbers of health care-related programs now available, at present the hospital trainer will not find enough commercially prepared programs for hospital-based educational needs, and those that are available may not meet the needs of a particular training situation. It may be a wise move to train a member of the hospital staff as a developer of self-instructional programs, who could be called upon for this purpose as needed, in addition to other regular duties. There are a number of academic and commercial sources offering training in the development and construction of self-instructional materials. The educator who knows how to develop programs also becomes better equipped to evaluate and select commercial programmed materials.

SELECTING TRAINING MATERIALS

The problem of selecting training materials is not confined to self-instructional programs. More than half of the respondents to the survey of hospital-based trainers indicated a need to learn more about creating training materials and evaluating packaged programs. M. Sue Pritchett, a specialist in educational materials, suggests the following checklist of five questions for the hospital-based trainer to ask himself as criteria for selecting commercially produced teaching materials or packages.[6]

1. *Are the objectives of the package spelled out in behavioral terms by the producer, and has the package been field tested?* If necessary, trainers should do their own testing and should communicate with the producer of the package if the results do not accord with the producer's claims.

2. *Is the total package specific to your training problem, or will you have to spend more time than is worthwhile adapting the package to your situation?* The trainer should particularly note whether the package was intended for groups, small teams, or individual learning.

3. *Is the material in a format you can use, and do you have the right equipment for it?* If the package is not compatible with the hospital's equipment, the trainer may inquire whether the material is available in another, more suitable format.

4. *Who is the author? Are you familiar with his work?* It is also helpful to ask others who have used the package how successful it was, and with what type of students.

5. *Is the cost of the package more than the cost of your training problem?* It is important to consider whether the material can be revised when training needs change.

PROPOSAL FOR AN INFORMATIONAL CLEARINGHOUSE

To make use of innovative methods and materials, an efficient national communications network is needed that will help educational planners and instructors in individual hospitals to become aware of new ideas and, especially, of available educational materials. It is economically inefficient for each trainer in a hospital to perform the necessary searches, particularly in view of the fact that some hospitals have as many as 200 occupational titles for which materials might be available. Such searches are often beyond even the capabilities of state or regional hospital associations. A national clearinghouse for educational materials would provide invaluable information to everyone engaged in hospital-based educational programming.

---

6. *Bulletin on Hospital Education and Training* (Chicago: Hospital Research and Educational Trust, October 1972).

The chief purpose of such a clearinghouse would be to identify, describe, and disseminate information on educational materials and publications in such areas as:

1. Correspondence courses for hospital personnel, encouraging greater use of such instruction

2. Periodicals and books in the field of continuing education, with particular attention to educational technology

3. Educational programs developed by commercial firms for the hospital market

4. Experimental continuing education programs developed by hospitals

5. Services of such agencies as the University of Rochester Clearinghouse, the Educational Resources Information Center (ERIC), the National Audiovisual Center of the National Library of Medicine, and so forth

6. Audiovisual software developed for hospital programs, with particular emphasis on the growing number of television tapes

The clearinghouse would not duplicate the activities of other agencies, but would function as the key transmission mechanism for informing the nation's health care institutions and organizations about the materials and publications available for training and continuing education.

9

Evaluating Continuing Education Programs

Everyone who is involved in hospital continuing education, whether in planning programs for national, state, or local hospital associations or for single hospitals or departments, needs to know the extent to which his efforts are productive of results on the job in the hospital, and he needs to know what should be done to make them more productive. Yet, with all of the effort—man-hours and dollars—expended over the years by hospitals and hospital associations on educational programming, it is unfortunate that so little effort has been spent in planning to meet specific objectives, or in evaluating the effect of all these short courses, seminars, institutes, and so forth. What is the anticipated or hoped for result of all this activity? Do those who conduct it really know? Do those who plan it really plan so that a meaningful evaluation can take place? Generally, the answer is no.

Evaluation may be considered the process of discovering whether, as a result of a given educational experience, a learner's behavior has changed in a desired direction. Behavior in this sense includes both cognitive or intellectual behavior (knowledge, understanding), which may be verified by verbal means, and overt behavior, which may be verified by observation. In other words, evaluation is a systematic process of measuring the results of an educational program against its objectives. If the objectives of the program have been framed in terms of the actual needs of hospital personnel, the process of evaluation will show to what extent those needs have been met.

Over the past several years, a number of experiments have been conducted in hospitals in which educational programs have been based on so-called "real needs"— as demonstrated, for example, by the review of medical records—rather than on the

85

"felt needs" of individuals or groups. From the national survey of trainers, it appears that most trainers are unfamiliar with, or inexperienced in using, techniques employing objective data for reliable determination of needs. However, it would seem that the objective approach, where applicable, would be in the long run the most rewarding course to follow for the improvement of patient care. Such an approach would lead to greater staff participation and to the kind of educational planning that is most relevant to the individual hospital.

As an intrinsic element of the interrelated activities of determining needs, establishing learning objectives, conducting programs, and measuring results, evaluation has been largely neglected in hospital continuing education. It is encouraging to note that the need to learn more about evaluating training programs carried out within their hospitals was given priority among their own needs by respondents to the 1972 survey of hospital-based trainers.

EVALUATING THE SHORT COURSE

Exactly what is meant by evaluation in the sense of a systematic process, beginning with program planning and carried on throughout a period of training? A brief discussion of the evaluation of the short course format in which hospital associations offer a large part of their continuing education programming may serve to illustrate the process. Both the coordinator of the short course and the hospital-based trainer who arranges for personnel to attend these courses need to determine their value to the participants and to the hospital.

In terms of a specific educational program, such as a short course or an institute, evaluation may be conducted in two phases: (1) evaluation of the participants' knowledge, understanding, or ability to do something as an immediate result of the educational experience, and (2) evaluation of the participants' change in behavior subsequent to the educational experience. The first phase involves evaluating the course by its instructional objectives; the second, evaluating the degree to which the course changed the participants' behavior on the job.

The steps in the process of evaluating a short course could be stated formally as follows:

1. Determine the objectives of the educational experience (determine what to evaluate).

2. Determine what specific behavior of the participants can be accepted as evidence of attainment of the objectives.

3. Determine the learning situations (methods and materials) that will stimulate the participants to exhibit the desired behavior.

4. Collect and record evidence.

5. Summarize the evidence and make judgments on the extent to which objectives have been met.

In actuality, of course, the specifying of objectives in behavioral terms and the planning of instructional procedures and situations form an organic activity. For example, consider an institute on planning that had three objectives: to give the participants knowledge and understanding of a planning process; to give them experience with a planning process; and to lead them to implement planning processes in the hospitals in which they were employed. The institute coordinator used reading assignments, lectures, and an actual case study for workshop discussions in order to provide learning situations to give the participants understanding of, and experience with, a planning process.

What specific behavior would demonstrate whether the first two objectives had been attained? Taking into consideration the subject matter, the participants, and the planned instructional procedures, the coordinator decided to ask the participants at the close of the institute to write about what they understood to be the steps of the planning process, to answer a written test in multiple choice or short-answer form, and to discuss with a workshop leader their understanding of planning. In fact, the coordinator made the workshop leaders part of a continuing process of evaluation throughout the institute. They were able to adjust the pace of their work groups and even to provide individual assistance or alternative learning experiences, as a result of their part in the evaluation.

To estimate progress toward the third objective—to have participants implement planning processes in their own institutions—the coordinator applied the second phase of evaluation, by following up in individual institutions. This phase was delayed so that the participants had time to implement a planning process in their own hospitals. Specifying the behavior to be observed seemed more difficult in this case, but the behavior was suggested by the content of the institute—for example, forming a planning committee. Evidence that changes of behavior were taking place was collected by a questionnaire mailed to participants, asking whether or not they were doing or had done specific things. Was a planning committee formed? Who were its members? When was it formed? The institute coordinator requested copies of records, or simple explanations of how planning was accomplished. The coordinator then had to decide whether the activity was actually in operation. After recording and summarizing the evidence, the coordinator of this institute was able to judge the extent to which participants had achieved the objectives, and the extent to which their learning experiences had been appropriate for realizing the objectives.

The actual process of evaluating a short course, or any other training program, may be difficult. It is necessary for the trainer to be explicit and precise in stating his objectives, and insofar as possible, to state them in behavioral terms. Because people are complex and always changing, it is difficult to measure their behavior, whether in terms of cognitive achievement or overt action.

In each phase of evaluation, the coordinator of a short course or institute, the hospital director of training and education, or the association director of education must be certain that the evidence he collects is worthwhile, and that it actually will measure understanding, or skill, or whatever behavior he is trying to teach. Records of evidence, whether in numerical or descriptive form, must be (1) objective—meaning that from the same set of records, another competent person would arrive at similar judgments about the extent to which goals have been attained; (2) reliable —meaning that the behavior recorded would be similar in another situation, under like circumstances; and (3) valid—meaning that the behavior observed and recorded was actually an example of the desired behavior.

It is best to use a combination of methods for evaluation. For example, to evaluate a program while it is in progress or immediately at its close, the trainer may ask the participants to complete a combination of tests or quizzes, rating scales, checklists, questionnaires, or inventories, to measure their achievements and attitudes. Other methods may be preferable for measuring the degree to which the participants' on-the-job behavior was changed or improved as a result of training. Among these are observation; interviews with the participants, their supervisors, and their co-workers; measurements of the quality and quantity of work performed before and after training; and review of pertinent records, such as records of patients' and employees' complaints, of accident rates, and of work attendance. Of course, the hospital-based trainer will find it easier to use these methods of on-the-job evaluation than will the outside coordinator of a short course.[1]

It is important, not only for trainers but especially for administrators and department managers, to understand that improved job performance depends on factors other than the quality of the training program or the achievement of the participants. Such factors include the circumstances of the work situation, and especially the attitudes and expectations of the participants' co-workers and supervisors. It is for this reason that evaluation of training is carried out in two phases: during or immediately after the training program, and later, in the work setting.

NEED FOR EVALUATION PROCEDURES

As in other educational areas in which the hospital field needs research, materials, and guidance, neglect in the area of evaluation unfortunately is reflected in a scarcity of assistance with evaluating continuing education programs, and of instruments for evaluating them, especially in the important second phase. Still, if the purpose of educational programming is to change behavior—to improve the effectiveness and efficiency of patient care—the only way in which success or failure can be judged and programming can be improved is by employing evaluation processes as an integral part of the training procedure.

For the students or participants, the process of evaluation provides a structured ending for their educational experience, motivating and reinforcing their learning.[2] For the trainer, the evaluation of any particular educational program yields evidence

---

1. For a full discussion of how to evaluate hospital training and education programs, including samples of data-collecting instruments, see Chapter 11, on evaluating results, in *Training and Continuing Education: A Handbook for Health Care Institutions* (Chicago: Hospital Research and Educational Trust, 1970), p. 221.

2. A report of the evaluation program that was carried out in conjunction with the management development course for administrators at Columbia University recommended involving students in both the planning and the evaluation of their educational experience, because this kind of involvement was found to motivate students by forcing them to make connections between their occupational and educational experiences. See Donna R. Barnes, "A report of the special testing and evaluation project for the management development course" (Center for Hospital Continuing Education, School of Public Health and Administrative Medicine, Columbia University, 1968).

of success in meeting the objectives, or evidence that suggests how the program may be revised and improved in light of the needs of the participants. From the point of view of the hospital administrator, as well as that of the director of training and education, evaluation is indispensable to obtaining reliable answers to questions about the value of specific educational commitments in relation to their costs.

If the objectives of a hospital or hospital association's total continuing education program have been developed from a careful study of the educational needs of hospital personnel, an evaluation of the entire program can provide evidence of the extent to which those needs are being met. For the field of hospital training and education as a whole, evaluation of every program is a necessary preliminary to communication among educators about successful model programs, curriculums, methods, and materials.

10

A Look Ahead

Energetic discussion is under way about restructuring the health care delivery system in the United States. Although public opinion focuses on the matters of access to the system and its financing, the need to continue providing the public with competent health care manpower is of equal importance if service of high quality is to result. The foremost purpose of continuing education is to enable hospitals and other health care institutions to maintain the competence and to improve the abilities of all those who work within them. To achieve this goal, health care manpower requirements must be identified, nationally and for given geographic areas, and regionally coordinated educational resources must be established, including universities, public educational systems, health planning agencies, health care providers, and those concerned with financing educational and health care services. Extending continuing education opportunities will be one of the major challenges to hospitals across the nation in the next several years, and the challenge will have to be met by nationwide effort and cooperation.

Although the hospital field still lags behind industry with regard to both the time and the resources devoted to continuing education, the progress made in the past few years has been striking. The academic community is becoming increasingly involved in the delivery of educational services to health care institutions. Regional, state, and metropolitan hospital associations are putting more resources into continuing education activities, many of which are designed to improve management skills and practices. A growing number of educational materials that utilize a variety of new technical aids are available from voluntary health care organizations and from commercial sources. There has been an absolute increase in the number of hospital personnel who plan and conduct continuing education and training, and an increasing number of these are directors of hospitalwide programs.[1]

Hospital administrators are coming to regard coordinated hospitalwide education as one of their principal strategies for improving manpower management and for keeping health care practices abreast of medical advances. Demands for additional hospital services are rising, along with pressures to contain hospital costs. It is becoming necessary for administrators to make major changes in organizing their human resources, because the manner in which personnel are managed has considerable impact on costs and on the effectiveness with which services are delivered. When used in the context of basic organizational and jurisdictional changes, continuing education can become a potent management tool, by means of which innovations are made acceptable and are integrated into the operating structure of the hospital.

Other problems arise from the accelerating increase in medical knowledge and the pace of technological change in the health care field. There is today a serious gap between available knowledge and its application in the delivery of health care services. Each member of the health care professions and each skilled hospital employee is threatened with the obsolescence of his knowledge and skills. At the same time, the need for better educated and more skilled labor continues to grow. Health care administrators who have not already designed and instituted educational systems to provide continuing education and training will need to do so, both to provide assistance to individual employees who need to update their training and to ensure the institution of having adequate skilled manpower.

EDUCATIONAL COMMITMENTS AND FINANCING

A decade ago, few hospitals offered hospitalwide continuing education opportunities, although hospitals have always been extensively committed to education. Today educational institutions—public school systems, community colleges, four-year colleges, and universities—are undertaking a large portion of the preservice education that prepares personnel for hospital employment. Still, clinical experience and education in the hospital remain indispensable, as does the hospital's participation in planning preservice education.

Hospitals also assume the primary responsibility for on-the-job training and for orientation of employees to the values, procedures, equipment, and physical facilities

---

1. In a national survey conducted in April 1973 by the American Hospital Association, the 5446 hospitals reporting (of 7182 surveyed) employed personnel who devoted all or part of their time to the coordination and delivery of inservice or continuing education for hospital staff. Of these, 9,668 were employed full time; 10,865, part time. In hospitals with fewer than 100 beds the ratio of part-time staff to full-time staff in educational activities was over four to one; in hospitals with 100 to 199 beds, the part-time/full-time ratio was reduced to five to four; and in hospitals with 200 beds or more, the ratio was reversed, with three full-time staff members for every two that were part-time.

Education departments were reported by 971 hospitals; they were staffed by 1898 full-time and 945 part-time educators and trainers. However, in 5103 hospitals nursing department personnel had some responsibility for coordinating and delivering inservice and continuing education; 6561 persons were involved full time and 6259 gave part of their time to this task.

of the health care institution. Although the final responsibility for continuing education rests with each individual health care worker, both professional and nonprofessional workers need opportunities for continuing education and assistance from the hospital in taking advantage of such opportunities. The same is true for all those engaged in management—supervisors, department managers, and administrators. The standards of the Joint Commission on Accreditation of Hospitals stipulate that hospitals shall provide, as one of their services, opportunities for the continuing training and education of health care personnel.

In addition, hospitals must develop the corporate commitment and the necessary resources for successful hospitalwide continuing education programs. A commitment to educational activities implies a commitment of financial resources. In addition to meeting the expenses of organizing and maintaining a program of continuing education and training, the hospital—as employer—should pay for the continuing education of its employees when it has requested or encouraged them to undertake training to improve their competency in their jobs. It is highly preferable for the hospital to fund its educational and training activities, insofar as possible, through nonoperating sources, such as tuition, scholarships, and private or public grants. Educational and training expenses that cannot be met through nonoperating funds must become the responsibility of all purchasers of health care.

PROFESSIONAL CONTINUING EDUCATION

A number of problems have arisen in regard to the continuing education needs of members of the health care professions. Basically, the continuing education of the health care professional is his own responsibility. On the other hand, to ensure patient care of high quality, hospitals—as employers—have a responsibility to see that physicians, nurses, and other members of the allied health professions avail themselves of continuing education opportunities. Health care educators and professional associations also have an interest in devising incentives that will ensure continuing professional education. The general public, as consumers of health care, are expressing the same interest, especially through their representatives in state legislatures and the Congress, and this interest is currently fueling a drive to make continuing education requirements mandatory in new laws for the periodic relicensing of health care professionals.

In 1972, the Commission on Medical Malpractice of the U.S. Department of Health, Education, and Welfare recommended that licensing boards in each state relicense physicians, dentists, nurses, and other allied health professionals on the basis of proof of compliance with standards for continuing education. The controversy that has arisen over these proposals stems from the observation that to mandate continuing education would be to lodge the primary responsibility for ensuring continuing education with state licensing boards, rather than with individual practitioners and their employers. Unfortunately, the past record of state licensing boards in the health care and other professions offers little ground for confidence that such a step is wise.

In the first place, state boards, which usually have fewer staff and less money than they need, are not qualified to assess the merits of the many experiences that may add up to valuable continuing education for a given individual. Clinical work experience; hospital-based refresher programs; non-credit institutes, workshops, seminars, and university extension courses; independent or self-directed study, using any of the media from books to tapes—all of these are difficult to measure and assess in quantitative terms, and they tend to be disregarded by licensing boards in favor of courses offered by traditional educational institutions for formal academic credit. This has been the practice of state boards in regard to initial licensing requirements, and also in regard to their decisions about the continuing education of nursing home administrators, which was required by an amendment to the 1968 Social Security Act. Secondly, because there is no uniformity of requirements among the state boards, reciprocal licensure would be difficult, inhibiting the movement of professional manpower from state to state.

Behind the demands for compulsory continuing education is the dubious assumption that participating in a given educational experience will automatically ensure improved performance. Otherwise, licensing boards would have to be empowered to evaluate job performance, to administer proficiency examinations, or possibly to prescribe remedial programs. To judge by past experience, boards would probably set general standards for the presentation of formal credentials, with little attention to the quality of actual performance on the job. Because of the difficulty of evaluating other forms of continuing education, the licensing boards and accrediting committees of professional associations also tend to demand formal academic credits or courses offered by the professional associations.

The touchstone for continuing education in its many forms must be quality of performance. National standards to measure the competency of professional and technical personnel should be developed or improved. Because in many instances credentialing methods have not kept pace with the changing roles, specialization, and expanded responsibilities of health care personnel, alternatives to existing licensure provisions should be identified, demonstrated, evaluated, and, if successful, adopted. It is essential for hospitals voluntarily to set standards of performance and to participate with professional associations and educational institutions in assessing the appropriateness of many kinds of continuing education, in appraising their results, and in improving the quality of nonacademic continuing education opportunities for the professional.

Professional education will be more effective if there is a plan for distributing learning periods throughout the working years, and if there is the opportunity to capitalize on special learning environments, both in the work situation and in educational institutions. The learning that takes place as the worker contributes to his professional organization is generally overlooked, but this, too, is surely continuing education. Studies of professional school graduates indicate that there are two important factors that determine whether the graduate maintains a high level of performance: (1) the attitudes and practices of colleagues with whom he maintains contact in his work, and (2) the availability of opportunities for continuing education to prevent deterioration of his performance.

Those health care professionals who are remote from urban centers or universities are especially in need of more accessible educational opportunities. The responsibility for creating more such opportunities in the future perhaps will lie in some new sort of cooperative effort by the hospital, a college or university in the region, and the professional associations.

The problem of obsolescence of knowledge and skills is especially acute in dealing with the return of inactive professionals to the hospital, and with the need—particularly in nursing—to rely upon part-time workers. Reentry of intelligent and highly motivated workers after temporary retirement, or the employment of such workers on a part-time basis, is always desirable. It is a difficult challenge to set up for such workers patterns of training that have both a sense of direction and continuity. Somehow, the funding agencies in vocational education must be persuaded to allocate the necessary financing for refresher training programs in health care. This, too, can be done only through a joint effort of national and state organizations.

A FINAL WORD: COOPERATION

Time is running out on the independent and uncoordinated efforts that have for too long been the hallmark of hospital and health care continuing education. For too long, there has been lip service to a fuzzily defined concept of the need for "life-long learning," without any significant coordination among the many health care agencies concerned with offering their share of it. Professional organizations, government agencies, trade associations, universities and colleges, and a variety of entrepreneurs have moved ahead, frequently oblivious of, or uninterested in, the work of others. Health care institutions pay large dues to support overlapping organizations that find it difficult to give up the prerogatives of autonomy and frequently duplicate one another's programs simply because they are strong enough to put together faculty and financing. There is lack of coordination at all levels—national, regional, state, and local. Effective coordination is difficult but not impossible to achieve; not to achieve it will be intolerable.

One wonders how long health care institutions—which frequently pay the expenses of registrants to attend meetings and short courses—will continue to foot the bill under these circumstances. The signs are that they are becoming impatient. In addition, state agencies are beginning to look at educational expenditures when they review institutional budgets, and to make decisions about how much an institution may allocate for such activities. The snail's pace at which the problem of how to rationalize and coordinate continuing education activities is being solved invites the increasing attention of such bodies to educational costs.

Some new partnerships are being hammered out locally among health care organizations and between health care organizations and educational institutions; but however worthwhile they may be in a given instance, they are too often the result of frustration and inability to determine a larger pattern into which they should fit. Sufficient instrumentalities already exist, and their mutuality of interest has been identified. What they must do is to begin a joint effort, commencing with work (not just dialog) at the national level, to define what those that have the largest resources of staff and money are uniquely equipped to do and are willing to do with some sense of commitment and continuity.

As Robert M. Hutchins, president of the Center for the Study of Democratic Institutions, has written, "Difficulties resulting from differences in background and vocabulary are stubborn, but not insuperable, and when they are overcome, a kind of light is thrown on the problem under study that no one of the participants could have generated for himself."

In the 1960s, it was essential not to chisel in granite a set of "thou shalts" and "thou shalt nots," but now, even while experimentation continues, tentative conclusions must be drawn as the basis for a program of joint action. Cooperative efforts are clearly the focus for the future.

APPENDIX A

Questionnaire for Hospital-Based Trainers

Please return by January 24, 1972, to:
HOSPITAL RESEARCH AND EDUCATIONAL TRUST
840 North Lake Shore Drive
Chicago, Illinois 60611

Survey of Members
AMERICAN SOCIETY FOR HOSPITAL EDUCATION AND TRAINING

Please refer to the mailing label above, answer the question below, and note any additions or corrections.

Is the information on the
above label correct?   Correction(s)

☐ Yes   _____

☐ No   _____

             _____

PERSONAL CHARACTERISTICS

1. Sex: ☐ Male   2. Age: ☐ Less than 25   ☐ 40 to 49

           ☐ Female   ☐ 25 to 29   ☐ 50 to 59

                                      ☐ 30 to 39   ☐ 60 years or more

3. If you are licensed, registered, certified, or accredited in some field,
    please check which, and specify field:

        ☐ License _____   ☐ Certificate _____

        ☐ Registration _____   ☐ Accreditation _____

4. If you possess one or more college degrees (associate, bachelor's, master's,
    doctorate, etc.), please specify the highest degree and the field in which
    it was earned.

        Highest Degree   Field in Which Earned

        ___ _____   _____

ORGANIZATION AND JOB CHARACTERISTICS

5. Are you employed by a health care institution?   ☐ Yes   ☐ No

    If "no," please answer a and b below.

    a. What is your job title? _____

    b. How does your work relate to health care? _____

        _____

    ┌──┐
    │ If you are not employed by a health care institution, PLEASE   │
    │ STOP HERE. The remaining questions are addressed only to   │
    │ trainers/educators in health care institutions.   │
    └──┘

6. What is the current size of your health care institution?

        ☐ Less than 100 beds   ☐ 300 to 399

        ☐ 100 to 199   ☐ 400 to 499

        ☐ 200 to 299   ☐ 500 beds or more

7. Does your institution have a separate department for hospitalwide training/
    education activities?   ☐ Yes   ☐ No

    a. What is the name of this department? _____

    b. What is the name of the department in which you are located?

    _____

8. Does your institution have a Director of Medical Education?   ☐ Yes   ☐ No

    If "yes," are your activities coordinated with his?   ☐ Yes   ☐ No

9. Are there other trainers/educators employed by your institution who devote
    half time or more to training and education? If so, please list their
    departments, their job titles, and their numbers.

Department	Job title	No. of persons
_____	_____	_____
_____	_____	_____
_____	_____	_____
_____	_____	_____
_____	_____	_____
_____	_____	_____

10. Is your current training/education position a full-time job?   ☐ Yes   ☐ No

    If "no,"

    a. What percent of your time do you spend on training/education?

                    ☐ Less than 50 percent

          ☐ 50 to 74 percent   ☐ 75 percent or more

    b. If your remaining time is spent in another department of your
        institution, please specify:

        Department _____ Job title _____

11. How many years were you employed in any job in the health care field before you assumed your current position?

☐ No previous experience

☐ Less than 1 year   ☐ 3 years but less than 5

☐ 1 year but less than 3   ☐ 5 years or more

> Please consider only your training/
> education job in answering the re-
> maining questions.

12. How many years of experience in a training/education role did you have prior to assuming your current position?

☐ No previous experience

☐ Less than 1 year   ☐ 3 years but less than 5

☐ 1 year but less than 3   ☐ 5 years or more

13. What is your current position title? _____

14. What is the position title of the person to whom you report?

_____   _____

15. At what organizational level is your position? That is, how many levels are there between you and the administrator? (If you report directly to him, check "none.")

☐ None

☐ One level   ☐ Two or more levels

16. How long have you held your current position with your present employer?

☐ Less than 1 year   ☐ 3 years but less than 5

☐ 1 year but less than 3   ☐ 5 years or more

17. How long has this position existed at your institution?

☐ Less than 1 year   ☐ 3 years but less than 5

☐ 1 year but less than 3   ☐ 5 years or more

JOB ACTIVITIES

18. Below on the left is a list of training/education needs. On the right below are
headings specifying methods for determining needs. For each need specified,
please check the method or methods that you yourself have used in determining the
need.

Training/Education Need	Interviews with administration	Interviews with department heads	Interviews with supervisors	Questionnaire surveys of employee groups	Work studies of employee performance	Records analysis (e.g., turnover)	Informal conversation	Other, specify below
New employee orientation								
Entry level skills training (please specify by job title; e.g., ward clerks or dietary aides)								
Continuing education (please specify by job title)								
"Refresher" training (please specify by job title)								
Upper management development								
First and second level supervisory development								
Medical staff continuing education								
Interdepartmental relations and coordination								
Community health education								
Patient education								
Basic literacy training								
English as a second language								
Other (please specify)								

Method Used To Determine Need

19. Below on the left is a list of training/education needs. For each item, place a check in the first column on the right if you yourself have planned a program to meet that need, and check the second column if you have actually conducted such a program. If these programs were for persons from more than one department, please also check the third column.

Training/Education Need	I Planned Program	I Conducted Program	Program Was Interdepartmental
New employee orientation	____	____	____
Entry level skills training (please specify by job title; e.g., ward clerks or dietary aides)			
_____	____	____	____
_____	____	____	____
_____	____	____	____
Continuing education (please specify by job title)			
_____	____	____	____
_____	____	____	____
_____	____	____	____
"Refresher" training (please specify by job title)			
_____	____	____	____
_____	____	____	____
Upper management development	____	____	____
First and second level supervisory development	____	____	____
Medical staff continuing education	____	____	____
Interdepartmental relations and coordination	____	____	____
Community health education	____	____	____
Patient education	____	____	____
Basic literacy training	____	____	____
English as a second language	____	____	____
Other (please specify)			
_____	____	____	____

20. Below on the left is a list of training/education needs. For each, please
     indicate whether you believe the need will change in your own institution
     during the next two years.

Training/Education Need	Increase	No Change	Decrease
New employee orientation	_____	_____	_____
Entry level skills training (please specify by job title; e.g., ward clerks or dietary aides)			
_____	_____	_____	_____
_____	_____	_____	_____
_____	_____	_____	_____
Continuing education (please specify by job title)			
_____	_____	_____	_____
_____	_____	_____	_____
_____	_____	_____	_____
"Refresher" training (please specify by job title)			
_____	_____	_____	_____
_____	_____	_____	_____
Upper management development	_____	_____	_____
First and second level supervisory development	_____	_____	_____
Medical staff continuing education	_____	_____	_____
Interdepartmental relations and coordination	_____	_____	_____
Community health education	_____	_____	_____
Patient education	_____	_____	_____
Basic literacy training	_____	_____	_____
English as a second language	_____	_____	_____
Other (please specify)			
_____	_____	_____	_____

21. Below on the left is a list of participant groups for whom you may have planned or conducted programs. On the right are headings describing various types of programs. Please indicate by check marks whether you yourself have planned (P) or conducted (C) such programs, for any of the groups listed, during the last 12 months (or since you began your job, if less).

Participant Group	Type of Program							
	Orientation		Skills Training		Continuing Education		Management Development	
	P	C	P	C	P	C	P	C
Administration								
Board of trustees								
Medical staff								
Department heads								
Business office								
Clinics								
Dietary/food service								
Housekeeping								
Laboratories								
Medical records								
Nursing, RN/LPN								
Nursing, other								
Volunteers (any age)								

22. Is your institution involved in conducting degree or certificate programs in cooperation with <u>educational institutions</u>? ☐ Yes ☐ No

If "yes," please check the kind(s) of institutions with which you are cooperating:

☐ University ☐ Vocational-technical school

☐ Four-year college ☐ High school

☐ Junior college ☐ Other (specify) _____

23. Are new cooperative degree or certificate programs now being planned for initiation during the next two years?

  ☐ Yes   ☐ No

If "yes," please check the kind(s) of institutions with which you will be cooperating:

  ☐ University   ☐ Vocational-technical school

  ☐ Four-year college   ☐ High school

  ☐ Junior college   ☐ Other (specify) _____

24. During the past 12 months has your institution been involved in cooperative (shared) programs with other hospitals and/or other health care institutions?

  ☐ Yes   ☐ No

If "yes," how many institutions other than your own were involved? _____

Please describe the trainees by job title or job level:

_____

_____

_____

_____

25. Are new cooperative programs with other health care institutions now being planned for initiation during the next two years?

  ☐ Yes   ☐ No

If "yes," how many health care institutions other than your own are involved? _____

Please describe the prospective trainees by job title or job level:

_____

_____

_____

_____

26. Below is a list of items that you may have used in programming. For those you have used during the past 12 months (or since you began this job, if less), please check the columns at the right to indicate whether the items were developed by you or your staff, or were commercially prepared.

Programming Item	Staff-developed	Commercial source
Educational TV (outside channels)		_____
Closed circuit TV	_____	_____
Slide-sound presentations	_____	_____
Filmstrips	_____	_____
Filmstrip-sound presentations	_____	_____
Transparencies	_____	_____
8mm movies	_____	_____
16mm movies	_____	_____
Tape recordings (audio)	_____	_____
Cassette tapes (audio)	_____	_____
Case problems	_____	_____
Demonstrations	_____	_____
Role plays	_____	_____
Training games	_____	_____
Action mazes	_____	_____
In-basket exercises	_____	_____
Sensitivity training exercises	_____	_____
Programmed instruction materials	_____	_____
Instructor's guides	_____	_____
Student manuals	_____	_____
Lesson plans	_____	_____
Evaluation questionnaires or rating forms	_____	_____
Other (specify)		
_____	_____	_____

27. Please indicate below whether, during the past 12 months, you have used the following as resource persons:

    Speakers/instructors from outside your institution?   ☐ Yes   ☐ No

    Consultants to assist with program development?   ☐ Yes   ☐ No

28. We would like to learn about specific features in your recent programs that you believe produced especially good results. Please identify these below. Include items of your own devising, as well as those commercially produced.

    _____

    _____

    _____

29. Below is a list of equipment. If an item is readily available to you at the present time, please put a check in the first column. If you plan to purchase it during the next two years, check the second column.

Item of Equipment	Now Available	Plan To Purchase
Overhead projector	_____	_____
Opaque projector	_____	_____
Slide projector	_____	_____
Filmstrip projector	_____	_____
8mm movie projector	_____	_____
16mm movie projector	_____	_____
Tape recorder (reel)	_____	_____
Cassette recorder	_____	_____
Cassette tape player	_____	_____
TV camera	_____	_____
Still camera	_____	_____
8mm movie camera	_____	_____
16mm movie camera	_____	_____
Slide-tape synchronizer	_____	_____
Videotape recorder	_____	_____
Videotape player	_____	_____
Other (please specify)		
_____	_____	_____
_____	_____	_____

30. Do your records show that over the past two years the funds available to you for training/education activities have:

☐ Grown significantly ☐ Been reduced significantly

☐ Grown somewhat ☐ Have no records

☐ Stayed the same ☐ Have no funds allocated to training/education

☐ Been reduced somewhat ☐ Other (specify) _____

31. If you were to have an "ideal budget," enough to meet all your training/education needs, what percent of that ideal budget would your actual current funds represent?

☐ Less than 10 percent

☐ 10 to 25 percent ☐ 51 to 75 percent

☐ 26 to 50 percent ☐ 76 to 100 percent

32. Below is a list of job components that may be relevant to your job activities. Please indicate the degree of influence you have over each of these job components.

Job Component	Degree of Influence			
	High	Moderate	Low	Not Relevant
Determining training and educational needs	___	___	___	___
Setting training and educational objectives	___	___	___	___
Determining content	___	___	___	___
Selecting speakers and instructors	___	___	___	___
Acquiring needed funds for activities	___	___	___	___
Selecting program participants or trainees	___	___	___	___
Developing programs to be carried out by others (including persons in other departments)	___	___	___	___
Supervising programs carried out by others	___	___	___	___
Evaluating the results of training and educational programs	___	___	___	___
Other (please specify)				
_____	___	___	___	___

33. Below is a list of various aspects of the trainer/educator's job. Please check those about which you would like to know more.

☐ Building learning principles into program designs

☐ Assessing training/education needs

☐ Setting measurable training objectives

☐ Creating tailored training materials (e.g., course outlines, workbooks)

☐ Combining elements of an educational program effectively

☐ Measuring training costs, as well as nontraining costs

☐ Achieving an effective instructional methods "mix"

☐ Evaluation of training/education programs within the institution

☐ Evaluation of packaged programs available from outside sources

☐ Other (specify) _____
_____

34. Below is a list of problems often encountered in training/education. Please check to indicate how much of a problem each of these items is to you.

Possible Problem	No Problem	Significant	Sericus
Not having enough qualified people to do the work	____	____	____
Not getting enough involvement on the part of higher management	____	____	____
Not getting enough cooperation from other departments	____	____	____
Not having enough outside resources available	____	____	____
Not having the knowledge or skills needed to carry out the work with confidence	____	____	____
Not having enough budget for needed materials, equipment, or facilities	____	____	____
Not having sufficient authority to make needed decisions	____	____	____
Other (specify)			
_____	____	____	____
_____	____	____	____

35. What aspect of your job as a trainer/educator was most rewarding to you during the past year? Please describe and explain.

_____

_____

_____

_____

_____

_____

_____

_____

_____

_____

_____

APPENDIX B

Questionnaire for Administrators

Questionnaire for Administrators on Their
Own Continuing Education Needs

1. Listed below are topics or content areas of possible interest to
   hospital administrators for their own continuing education.

   A. In Column A please check the content areas in which you have had
      continuing education in the last two years (apart from your in-
      dividual reading).

   B. In Column B please number content areas in order of interest to you,
      to indicate areas in which you personally would like continuing
      education. Please mark your priorities from 1 to 5, with number 1
      indicating your highest priority and number 5, your lowest.

Content Area	A Content Areas Studied in Last Two Years	B Content Areas Ranked in Order of Priority
Design and Construction		
Economics		
Education and Training		
Financial Management		
Fund Raising		
Governing Board Relations		
Institutional Planning		
Legal Developments		
Management Engineering		
Medical Staff Relations		
Organizational Theory		
Personnel Administration		
Psychology		
Sociology		
Other (please indicate)		

2. Listed below are different types of sources for continuing education.

    A. In Column A please check the sources that you have used during the last two years.

    B. In Column B please check which of these sources you would prefer to use in meeting the continuing education needs you have indicated in Column B of Question 1.

Sources	A Sources Used in Last Two Years	B Sources Preferred if Available
CLASSROOM PROGRAMS Institutes or Other Short-Term Programs .		
University or College Evening Courses . .		
INDIVIDUAL READING Books		
Journals.		
Newsletters		
SELF-INSTRUCTIONAL MATERIALS Audio cassettes		
Correspondence Courses.		
Television.		
OTHER Conventions		
Sabbatical Leaves for Advanced Study. . .		
Study Tours		
Additional Sources Used (please specify).		

3. Please indicate any additional recommendations you care to make regarding education of executives with experience comparable to your own.

_____

_____

_____